Medical Mayhem

Dee Mitchell

[handwritten signature]

VANTAGE PRESS
New York

To patients, medical professionals, and friends

Published by Vantage Press, Inc.
516 West 34th Street, New York, New York 10001

Manufactured in the United States of America
ISBN: 0-533-11545-0

Library of Congress Catalog Card No.: 95-90340

0 9 8 7 6 5 4 3 2 1

Contents

Introduction

There were only a handful of female plastic surgeons in 1960 when I began my private practice. After over fifteen years of university, medical school, internship, general surgery residency, and plastic surgery preceptorship, it was a new outlook to see my name, Dee Mitchell, M.D., Plastic and Reconstructive Surgery, on the office door. That door opened into a space so small it could have been a converted mouse hole.

Some years would pass before there was another woman practicing in the state, and it was three years before my husband, Armando, joined me in the office. During those three years I worked alone or with physicians of other specialties, caring for the middle class, the migrants, and the millionaires with results that were sometimes thought provoking, sometimes hilarious, occasionally bizarre, and at other times tragic.

The millionaires lived on the barrier island across the intracoastal waterway, the middle class in a four-block-wide strip between the intracoastal and the railroad, the Negroes (so called then) lived west of the tracks, and the migrants wherever they could out in the mucklands of the Everglades.

These vignettes were gleaned from those twenty-three years, also earlier times and other encounters along the way. Many involved Armando, schooled both in Latin America and the USA, with the resultant cultural and language ships that tended to collide rather than pass in the night.

Statistics

"It'll be a snap, just as easy as pie, no trouble at all." Harry's pronouncement was delivered with his usual conviction, which tended to be in inverse proportion to the realities. His jaunty step and bright plaid shirt marked the eternal optimist. I took a dim view of it and told him so.

"Harry, where judgment is concerned, you are one of the walking wounded. The bottom line on your commonsense balance sheet is in red ink."

He gave a devil-may-care shrug and tossed his blond hair back from his forehead as his bright blue eyes shone with optimism and he accused me of being a perennial pessimist.

We were on our way to a seminar each of us needed for its one hour of upper-division science credit. It involved the mathematics and science departments and seemed easy enough. The one hour of weekly attendance was mandatory; in addition, each participant had to present a paper.

I'd been working on mine for several weeks. Being in organic chemistry I'd seized on the possibilities of the urea molecule, tracing the metabolic changes possible as it was formed and excreted. It wasn't a really great paper but probably adequate for a B+.

Harry was in genetics and busy breeding fruit flies. The color of their eyes follows the laws of heredity like the peas of the monk Mendel. That puts it as badly as I had done when I'd taken the class. My flies had wakened from their anesthesia and flown off before I could get the microscope focused, so

1

maybe I was unfairly casting doom and gloom on Harry's enterprise.

Harry burbled on in his prefrontalized enthusiasm. "I saw on the bulletin board that today's seminar is by one of those stodgy mathematics types. He's going on about the statistical analysis of small samples. All I'll have to do is take down his formulas, apply them to my fruit flies, and presto, there's my seminar for presentation."

As we entered the building, I gave him my grim verdict. "You're barking up a a leafless tree, my friend, but good luck in your landing when you fall out of it."

Harry sat in the front row, all attentiveness, and copied formulae from the blackboard. The math type droned on about laws of probability, which had always been an enigma to me. Next he got into some calculus and my background in that was minimal so I watched Smith, a graduate student who was grading papers in the next-to-the-last row.

My attention wandered farther when Marcy, sitting beside me in the last row and doing the daily paper's crossword puzzle, gestured for my help. She needed the word for a six-carbon ring-structured molecule. She, too, had no interest in small-sample analysis. Her field in physics was light and wavelength transmission, which didn't come in analyzable small samples.

Finally the minute hand of the clock inched toward the hour and the more somnolent participants began to stir. In a triumphal grand finale, the mathematician delivered his miraculous message: "To do a statistical analysis of a small sample, divide it into even smaller samples."

And there sat Hopeful Harry in the front row, with sheets of paper covered with formulae, while back in his lab, waiting to be divided into smaller samples for analysis, was his small sample—a single fruit fly with apricot-colored eyes.

The Locked Cupboard

Sister Barbara was usually all business, the starched white skirts of her "on duty" habit swishing briskly as she patrolled her domain. Although no longer young, she had much more empathy for the student nurses than most of the nuns exhibited. No word was ever said about it, but she seemed to understand our weariness with the constant bread, beans, macaroni, and potato diet to which we were subjected.

During the war, when sugar was rationed, every patient received a tiny paper nut cup of sugar on their tray with each meal. Before the trays were returned to the kitchen in the basement, Sister Barbara quickly and deftly removed all of the unused sugar and put it into an empty two-pound coffee can, which she kept in her locked cupboard behind the chart desk. We did not dare question her actions but sometimes wondered what became of the sugar.

Finally, early one afternoon, she gave everyone special work to keep them busy. Two students were sent with extra drawsheets and pillowslips to recheck all of the potentially incontinent patients. One girl had to scrub down and do special housecleaning in the nurses' lavatory—washing lightbulbs and all those little things that seldom were accomplished in our foreshortened time frame. The old wing, unheated, gloomy, and long closed, was to be reopened. Military dependents and war workers flooding into the area had overwhelmed the facilities of the new building. Sister

Barbara found this an excellent time to send four students to scrub walls and ceilings in preparation for painting.

She sent Helen to the kitchen with a note for the nun who was in charge of that domain. Helen returned with a closed sack, which she gave (unexamined of course) to Sister Barbara. I was detailed to go into the back portion of the linen closet to mend some of the nuns' habits. All of the junior students were resentful of the extra work. I wasn't. I liked sewing better than working on the wards. The senior student on duty was kept at the chart desk to do chartwork and answer lights. Sister Barbara locked herself in the little serving kitchen.

Presently, enticing odors began to sneak out from under the door, and we knew then what the sack had contained. At the change of shifts, Sister Barbara surprised all of us with a pan of fudge well laced with filbert nuts. One of the patients of our sister hospital in Portland had paid part of his account in produce from his nut orchard. Speaking on behalf of all of us, Sister Barbara intoned, "Praise be!"

That fudge treat continued, sugar supply permitting, during the war, but it wasn't Sister Barbara's only foray into her locked cupboard for our benefit.

In late January we had a private-duty nurse, a Mrs. Frampton, caring for a patient on our floor. He was an aged and undemanding patient, who spent most of his time asleep. This nurse was a rather mentally and emotionally constipated type. If there was a narrow view of a subject to be had, she would ferret it out and espouse it. She was WCTU (Women's Christian Temperance Union): antismoking, antitrousers for women, antipermanent waves, and anti any kind of enjoyment.

While we were all bemoaning the lack of sweets in our diet one day, she rather hesitantly said, "I've part of a Christmas fruitcake left over, but it's so dry I'm embarrassed to offer it to you."

Sister Barbara pounced on what she chose to interpret as an offer. "You just bring it right in tomorrow and I'll show you how to remoisten it with an apple."

The next day Mrs. Frampton brought in three-fourths of a huge fruitcake. It was full of pecans, walnuts, marachino cherries, pineapple, and all sorts of other goodies. A kind of relative of Mrs. Frampton's who was in the military had sent it from a PX. Sister Barbara made a great show of cutting a raw apple into eighths and wrapping cake and apple carefully in waxed paper.

"Now," she said "in a few hours, when the cake is a little softer, it can be sliced without crumbling and rewrapped." With that pronouncement she unlocked her cupboard and placed a tray with the large packet reverently within.

Patients' trays were passed at 5:30, and immediately thereafter, all of the other nurses left to go to supper. Sister Barbara and I were to "keep the floor" for the half an hour they would be gone.

Sister Barbara wasted no time. She beckoned me from behind the chart desk, quickly unlocked her cupboard, motioned me to hunker down on the floor where I couldn't be seen, and had me cradle the cake in my hands. Her starched habit crackled as she whirled back to the shelf; then, from behind the cupboard door, she hastily poured a number of generous dollops of liquor from a pint bottle into the cake.

Sister outlined the drill for me then. "Just before you go off duty, I'll be back from chapel and we'll slice this confection. During the years before the war when we still had janitorial help, Father Bennigan's private supply vanished regularly during the hour he was in chapel saying mass so he asked me to keep it in my locked cupboard, knowing no one else had a key. Now here it has paid its own rent."

Next afternoon Mrs. Frampton was practically jubilant at the miraculous manner in which her donation had been rejuvenated. All of the nurses were happy too, but being more worldly and knowing liquor when they smelled it, were a bit more subdued in their praise of the apple.

As the end of her shift approached, Mrs. Frampton became more fulsome and tended to squeal a bit about the whole business as she snatched another mouthful, which she called "a tiny, delicious crumb."

Suppertime came and the other nurses left the floor, leaving Sister Barbara and I alone again.

"Now you run up the backstairs with this generous slice of cake for Father Bennigan. It will serve as a sort of thank offering to Providence, whose ways, you will observe, Miss Mitchell, are sometimes peculiarly inscrutable.

The Sleds

Marian and I couldn't really complain that Sister Michael had sneaked up on us. She never did let her beads rattle as the other nuns did.

Maybe they couldn't rattle anyway. She made them herself, sometimes with our conscripted assistance. It was a good thing that the Oregon coast was ideal rose-growing country as rose petals were scrounged from everyone she knew and probably as many that she did not know. The petals were ground up, rolled into small cylindrical masses, dried, drilled, and wired together with fine surgical wire. They carried forever the faint scent of a rose garden in the summer sun.

We often marveled at how out of character it seemed for Sister Michael to make something with a scent so subtle. Subtlety and Sister Michael were total strangers. She and Sister Johanna, head of the nurses' training school, were martinets. It was rumored that they were related and for sure they shared a Teutonic obsession with precision in work and speech.

This was manifest in the manner in which Sister Michael gave us our surgical training. Arriving on rotation, the student was bidden to completely houseclean the entire surgery and redo and resterilize all the surgical packs. Then, as she sat on a tall stool in the workroom, Sister Michael would interrogate the student about the location of a certain pack: Which shelf? Between which other packs? Below and above which packs? The student also had to enumerate the contents of the pack. Then the viewpoint would change, and the student would be grilled as to what was on such and such a shelf, in room number so and so, between the appendectomy tray and incision and drainage pack. Sister Michael seemed to feel that a person had to be destroyed and remolded to be a proper surgical nurse. She impressed upon each one that a life might ebb away while a nurse frittered her time away looking for something important.

Sister Michael didn't like me. I had, at that age, a photographic memory, which in her mind was an evil, devilish thing—something ungodly, like cheating. Further, no matter how abusive she became, I would never cry. Fighting my way through a childhood with thirteen little boys and no girls had taught me that crying was self-destructive.

It was fine with me that she didn't like me. I didn't like Sister Michael either. Bullies were things to be scorned. We did, however, have a certain appreciation for each other's abilities, and even then I had a sneaking feeling that in future years her teachings would save my bacon more than once.

All that is beside the point. Marian and I were on surgery rotation and were sitting on the tall stools in the workroom. It was in 1941, when those things were still done, and we were patching surgical gloves. As we did, we talked quietly about the delights of sledding as children. The matter had arisen as we peered through the falling snow toward the hill outside the window, where two Red Flyer sleds were coasting down the hill then being towed back up again by their trudging little passengers, who were all muffled up in scarves, mittens, and galoshes.

It was a rare treat for them. Winter there at the mouth of the Columbia River was cold and raw for days on end, the icy rain driven up the gorge by a ravening wind. Snow in any quantity was rare though, and the children were making the most of it.

Marian and I fell silent as Sister Michael appeared in the

doorway. She did not hold with meaningless chatter and made it clear that speech unrelated to our work or matters religious was very unwelcome. Sister walked over to the window, looked out through the swirling powdery snow, then left the room without a word. It was nearly her dinnertime so we supposed she had left the floor, and after a few minutes we continued our conversation.

We were really taken by surprise when she appeared again at the door and announced that she had just spoken to the mother of the two children, who she knew from her summertime rose collecting. "The children have gone in for the night, and if you hurry, you will have three-quarters of an hour before your dinner to go sliding. I have every hope that it will sweep the cobwebs from your heads. I will keep the surgery while you are gone. When you have finished with the sleds, dry them carefully and put them on the drip mat just inside the convent door. The children will get them in the morning."

On our way to get the sleds, Marian and I marveled at Sister Michael, who usually seemed almost sadistic. How many times had I seen girls crying as they scrubbed for surgery, while she berated them from the doorway of the room containing the scrub sinks. We discussed her apparent need to destroy a person's spirit, somewhat in the manner of the man who beats a horse or dog to "train" them.

On the hill we had a grand time flushing "the cobwebs" from our heads. Being carefree and childish again was a marvelous relief from our strictured and structured existence, and it enabled us to face the inevitable supper of macaroni and beans with reddened faces and equanimity instead of our usual whispered carping.

I had left the autoclave on, sterilizing some of the smaller surgical packs, and had to leave the table before my suppertime was officially over. On the way up the stairs (we were forbidden to use the elevators), a glance out the window assured me that a few lazy flakes of snow still drifted down. They weren't enough, though, to obscure the activity on the hill. Flying full tilt downward on the little sleds were two figures, their black habits streaming, whirling, and twisting with the speedy descent.

Later, Sister Michael came by the surgery for a last check before bedtime. "And did you find, Miss Mitchell, that the exercise and fresh air swept the cobwebs from your brain?"

"Indeed, I found that it did, Sister Michael. Did *you* not find it so as well?"

An extremely brief and fleeting unguarded expression of a cornered animal was replaced immediately on Sister Michael's face by her usual uncompromising aspect as she turned, wordless, to glide down the hall toward the elevator.

Never again when I was in the surgery did she try to reduce the nurses to tears for I was in a position to deliver the ultimate humiliation.

I knew, and she knew that I knew, she was human.

Fleas

We had only one "secure" room in the hospital. It had bare floors, barred windows, the whole bundle of wax.

It was inevitable that I would be assigned to care for Tom Neeny. I'd always been almost pathologically strong for my age and sex, and growing up in a neighborhood of numerous boys and no other girls had honed my instincts for self-preservation.

Tom, they told us, had been living in an old chicken coop in an abandoned farm back in the hills. The other buildings had long since burned and sagged back to the earth with the help of the ever-present Oregon "mist." How he found any food for his two mangy, scruffy curs after he'd paid for the makings of the lifeline to put in his still, no one knew. Maybe the dogs hunted meat for him as well as themselves.

One black rainy night in the early years of World War II, Tom was lurching along the secondary road about three miles from his habitation when he was hit by a military vehicle. The Coast Artillery were out on night maneuvers, and, of course, that was during the years of a total blackout there on the coast.

A combination of head injury, rotgut whiskey, and probable internal injuries landed him in the small hospital where I was a second-year nursing student.

Doing my best to care for the man, who was somewhat violent at times and had minor seizures at others, didn't bother me. Trying to get him to eat without being attacked with a fork or knife was okay too. Somehow the kitchen couldn't get it through their thick heads that "finger food" should be just that.

In those years, we worked split shifts, and to be truthful, very little was accomplished for Neeny when I wasn't there. The other nurses were afraid of him with his filthy, tangled hair and wild, darting gaze. The floor nun excused herself from the situation because "his language is so foul."

After two days, some bit of cleanliness was beginning to show. I'd snipped off some of his hair while he was distracted with food, but the situation was taking its toll on me in other ways. However, being short on doctors and nurses, with no janitorial staff and no orderly, we were taught to be resourceful, self-reliant, use our common sense, and not complain.

Finally I took my bundle of woes to Sister Paul of the Holy Name, the directress of the nursing school. Before knocking on the door of her office, I quickly checked the condition of my hair, uniform, shoelaces, and shoes.

"Enter." Sister Paul's voice was as devoid of inflection as her office was of nonessentials. Standing before her plain desk behind which she sat on a straight chair, I couldn't help thinking that the picture of Christ above her head had probably been painted by an artist who looked down his nose at humanity, just as Sister Paul was looking at me—with disinterest if not disdain.

Not wishing to prolong the encounter, I stated my case. "Sister Paul, I need some help."

"And what is it, Miss Mitchell, that you cannot manage for yourself?"

It occurred to me that she would have sneered if such an action had been permitted her, but I spoke up anyway. "It's not entirely for me. I've been caring for Mr. Neeny in the security room for six days now."

"Yes." It wasn't a question. She was immobile and her face

12

expressionless. I could see she had really no interest in my problems and was not going to make things easy for me.

"I'm not getting much sleep and am late for classes. Twice a day when I get off duty, I have to shower, shampoo my hair, and boil all my clothes. The patient was alive with fleas and who knows what other vermin when he was brought in. I've done my best and he's cleaned up some, but the room is still a crawling, leaping mess. He's a little calmer but not much, and he's not trustworthy yet. You can't turn your back on him because he's still manic at times and frequently won't take the medication that would calm him a bit."

The nun spoke. "Have you, Miss Mitchell, prayed about this problem?"

All of a sudden I was too tired and fed up with the situation to contain myself, so I stared her straight in the eye and answered her back.

"Yes, I did, Sister John Paul. While I was on my knees at prayers, some of the fleas leaped on the other girls and distracted all of us. Despite that, I did receive an answer to my prayers."

For the first time her face showed some fleeting interest. "And what answer did you receive?"

"An inner voice told me very distinctly to consult my superior, so here I am."

Sister John Paul looked right through me, eyes focused on the far past, the days perhaps when she was still hopeful for the ecstasy so many of the religious expect and so few attain. For the first time ever, I saw her face soften.

She spoke. "I acquired vermin from a patient once many years ago—just after taking my final vows."

Surely, I thought, a quick and final solution would be forthcoming now. Just think about fleas in those voluminous wool habits and convoluted starched coifs. Anyone who could manage that situation could certainly tell me in a few words

13

how to control it with clothes that were at least washable. That would leave only the twice daily shampoo of my long, thick hair, which stayed damp in the Oregon climate from one washing to the next.

Excitedly I moved one step forward and asked urgently, "What did you do about them?"

Her expression as stony as ever, Sister John Paul stood and with one word disposed of my problems, Mr. Neeny and his fleas, and terminated our interview.

"Scratched."

Dammit Johnny

Sister John was in her midseventies during the years of the Second World War. She had entered the order at about age sixteen, trained as a nurse, and spent almost all of her life on night duty. Put that way, it sounds pedestrian enough, but Sister John was mortally afraid of the dark.

This made the whole business of night duty a penance for us. She wouldn't leave the area of the chart desk (which was blacked out so we barely had enough light for desk work) and had an uncanny knack for putting her rocker where we had to stumble over her to answer call bells. Our only relief came when she finally screwed up enough courage to go to the chapel to say her prayers. That wasn't often as the chapel was on an upper floor of the old building, reachable by a long black corridor and fearsome dark stairs. More often she retreated to the nurses' lavatory, which was very near us and had no windows. Or, if the first room next to the chart desk happened to be empty, she would hie herself thence. We could hear the squeak of her rocker on the terrazzo floor and the soft clatter of her rosary beads until these sounds were supplanted by gentle snores.

We called her "Dammit Johnny," even to her face. She didn't dare complain. It would have been an admission that we'd been getting away with it. Being asked to shampoo her hair in the middle of the night when everything was going wrong—a difficult labor in the delivery room, dying patients at opposite ends of the hall, and the local lush screaming that

15

little green men with spinning eyes were jumping on him from the bedrail . . .

Dammit Johnny was, in a word, exasperating.

This particular night, we had just sent the family of one of the dying patients to the hotel for a much-needed rest after their long bus trip from three states away. We'd promised to let them know at once if he came out of his coma or if there was an abrupt deterioration in his condition.

Suddenly, in the middle of my charting, I had that urgent feeling that there had been a change in his situation. Night duty especially, if you let it, will hone your intuition to a fine edge.

Jumping up and stumbling over Johnny, her beads, and her rocker, I raced down the hall and into the patient's room. Even with the feeble light cast by a flashlight covered with red cellophane, it was apparent that some ghastly terminal event was under way. The patient's color was dark, despite convulsive gasping. I thought it probably was a pulmonary embolus—a clot that had floated from his long unused legs into his lungs. It was very evident that there was no time to get morphine to relieve him or do anything else but throw open the window and hope the fresh air would ease his last few breaths.

Turning back from the window to the bed, I was just in time to see Dammit Johnny reaching over the side rails to shake the poor fellow violently and yell at him, "Say Jesus save us! Say Jesus save us!"

By this time my patience with her was exhausted. I reached across the bed, gave her a shove, and spoke sternly. "Dammit, Johnny, shut up and let the poor devil die in peace."

Johnny gave a startled gasp and scuttled off down the hall, her beads beating a rapid tattoo.

The necessary formalities of a death had to take precedence over the apology I knew I owed the nun and intended to give as soon as possible. The family, the physician, and the mortician had to be notified first; then the chart had to be closed and the patient's personal effects bagged to send with the body, which we took to the morgue in the hospital basement.

In the end she beat me to the draw. When Dammit Johnny returned from her early private prayers in the chapel, apparently she either felt she had misjudged my efforts and intentions or perhaps she had glanced at the chart. If she had done that, she may have realized that screeching, "Say Jesus save us!" was neither productive nor appropriate for one whose name was Saul Finkelstein. Gliding up to stand beside me, she offered her version of an apology. "I must admit, Miss Mitchell, you can always tell when they are going to die."

The Motive

Agatha tended to be more religious or "churchy" than I was, so when her strident voice bounced back in an aggressively belligerent sort of way from the low gable ceiling with a pronouncement of finality, "It's a flat-out miracle, I tell you," I heard it with only one ear.

"What's a miracle?" I asked to be polite, all the while paying major attention to juggling hot tea, knitting, and a neuroanatomy book. The tea slopped, but minimally.

"That this blasted sieve of a barn that Pop Dean calls a house hasn't collapsed in on itself long ago and floated from Portland down the Columbia River into the Pacific."

She was right, of course. Pop had built it himself on the edge of a barranca. Even the shift in one corner of the foundation couldn't explain the four-inch deviation from a square corner when I'd laid a linoleum remnant over the rough boards of a five-by-nine-foot closet, which did its meager duty as my bedroom. If Pop hadn't been so kind to the struggling medical and physiotherapy students, we'd all have left the battleship gray–painted woodwork and floors behind long ago. It was, however, the cheapest place to live on the medical school hill, and it was a hard scratch to come up with even the modest rent he asked, so there we sat in the draught that poured cold Oregon damp under the doors and around the windows. Our legs were wrapped in quilts, the tea warmed our hands as we held the cups, and the knitting helped to keep them from being too stiff to turn the pages.

"Whatever are we doing here anyway—making modern martyrs of ourselves?" Agatha's question had more than a note of defiance.

I picked at some frayed threads from the arm of the davenport and reflected a moment before answering.

"Can't speak for you, but I'm here because law seemed a dusty way to go, my loathing for math eliminated engineering, and a total lack of talent for any facet of it left out architecture. By taking three years of nurses' training I thought I could work nights and, hopefully, put myself through medical school. It really seemed the path of least resistance. I don't want to spend my life taking orders from people dumber than I am." What little I knew about Agatha's family told me that graduate-level schooling wasn't part of their expectations for a girl, so mild curiosity prompted me to ask, "And you?"

Anger against the fates flared in her chill blue eyes and a blue vein distended up the middle of her forehead. "Dad was a maintenance man on the machinery in the pulp mill. When the depression came, paper wasn't selling so the mill closed down. Mom had never worked and had no salable skill. Dad odd-jobbed what there was, but with my two brothers and I to clothe and feed, things were pretty thin. Mom could sew basic things and that helped. When the neighbors gave her limp leftover celery, carrot, and potato peelings intended to feed our chickens, she used them to make soup for us. We kids scavenged weed seeds and tender young weeds for the chickens. One of the catastrophes of that time was when a hawk took one of our few aging hens."

Agatha shook her long, wavy brown hair and hitched her quilt tighter around her feet and legs, bundled her teacup momentarily in her hands, then continued.

"The summer after I finished eighth grade there was a fledgling mint industry started there in the Willamette River valley; acres of mint and a mint press—the whole bit. I got a job there and spent six days a week on my hands and knees weeding the mint beds. At the end of the summer there was enough money for a blouse, a skirt, a sweater, a pair of saddle oxfords, a change of underwear, and two pairs of bobby socks. Absolute riches! This went on for two more years, then pfft."

"Did they quit growing mint or what?" I asked, thinking the mint would have given a welcome boost to the third cup of hot water I was pouring over the same teabags.

Agatha jabbed her knitting needle viciously into the stiff bargain-basement yarn. "The Monday after school was out I packed my lunch, put on my old clothes, and went confidently out to the mint field. The owner waved me off airily and announced, 'We don't need you. We've found that a flock of geese will eat everything but the mint when the weeds are too small to pull by hand. They don't cost us a dime either.' And with that, he took his smug face back to the barn.

"There's nothing like that for motivation, I tell you. Here I was, practically at the end of what I perceived as my formal education, and it was flung in my face that I could be replaced—and advantageously—by a goose."

Oncology

Oncology wasn't a very well-developed specialty in the late 1940s and early 1950s. About all we could do for cancer patients was operate, give X-ray therapy, prayers, and morphine.

The one class we had, therefore, wasn't conducted as the usual didactic lecture. Students were put into clusters of three or four and were told to prepare a paper for presentation to the class on some aspect of malignant tumors. Each group could select their own topic.

With the exception of one other class, this was the only time in my four years of medical school that I worked with other women. There were only five of us in the class, and three of us were assigned to work together on the project, which we decided would be on cancer quacks.

Mary was the oldest and, with white hair at her temples, the most credible candidate for a cancer patient. Moreover, her husband was a businessman and she taught at the medical school, so she could afford to be the guinea pig. She was to go from one to another of the people who advertised cancer cures and relate classic symptoms of a malignancy then report what happened and how, exactly, they proposed to "cure" her. Mary was quiet, introspective, and a great listener, her gray eyes fixed on the speaker's face. We saw her as a near-middle-aged lady, who was short, serious, shy, and unsmilingly scholarly. As a matter of fact, she was our instructor in physiologic chemistry, having a doctorate in that discipline.

I was to research the literature and popular magazines for all the material I could find on well-known cancer quacks. Laura would organize the lot and put it all together in a paper.

Usually Mary didn't join the traditional coffee group in the cafeteria early in the morning, but it was the most convenient time for the three of us to meet and exchange the results of our efforts. Soon other medical students found out what was happening and joined us for a blow-by-blow of Mary's latest effort.

One of her first expeditions was to an Oriental gentleman, who held forth as an herbalist down near the waterfront. Retiring by nature, it wasn't easy for Mary to be passing winos leaning on doorjambs of shuttered, extinct businesses, but she gave us a full report of her first visit on a Monday.

As she spoke, I could see her pulling her scarf tight around her face, scuffing through all the papers and debris that eddied in the recessed doorways. At first, she said, she had worried about what the Chinese gentleman thought of her. A wad of discarded gum had stuck to her shoe and fatally attracted a portion of urine-stained newsprint. "I thought he would laugh at me, thinking I was a handicapped duck," she said, "but that notion was immediately superseded by a fascinated horror at my surroundings. The one-hundred-year-old musty, dusty, haymow smell in the dingy place gave me the urge to flee precipitously."

Before she could even turn around, she reported, a late-middle-aged Oriental man started chattering and never really stopped. Somehow she levered in a few words about symptoms, rapid weight loss, coughing blood, etc. The fellow fished out some old dusty jars from equally dirty shelves. Brushing the cobwebs off, he put some leaves from each into a scrap of ancient yellowed newspaper, twisted the ends together, and kept repeating, "Make tea, make tea, make tea." By this time, Mary was so numb with alarm that his addition of the bill on his abacus didn't even startle her. It was $5.40. As she hastened to escape, her gummed foot retarding her progress, he was twittering after her, "Drink many times in day. Come back one week, Missus."

While Mary was communing with her Oriental specialist, I was busy summarizing articles on the use of the powers of the pyramids known by the ancients. One wonders, if they were that knowledgeable, why their life expectancy was so brief. Short shrift was given to the East Indian guru who proposed (for a fee of course) to do an authentic deciphering for me. Then there was a man broadcasting to the Midwest from a radio station just across the border in Mexico. He implied that all urinary and reproductive functions of men over a certain age were cancerous and that he alone possessed the secret of successful treatment *without surgery* (this last shouted in a startling voice). Also implied was the idea that the delicacy of the matter precluded public announcement of exactly how this was to happen.

Before briefing us the next time we met for coffee, Mary slipped out of her raincoat, hung it neatly over a chair, and retrieved a handful of tissues from the pocket. Wearily she pushed her simply cut hair from her forehead with the back of her hand and dabbed gently at her raw red nose with one of the tissues. Her eyes were red and swollen, and her voice flat and rough from the stuffiness in her head. She had been off to a religious faith healer, and they had gone together at midnight to the Morrison Bridge over the Willamette River. Mary had, she said, given the woman the symptoms of a uterine malignancy. "And there we were," she went on, "she was praying away, really howling against that cold wind, shrieking for that tumor to drop away into the river. I tell you that icy blast up under my clothes would have chased any self-respecting cancer back into the warmth it had left." Mary coughed, blew her nose, took a sip of her hot brew, and continued. "That cost me twenty-five dollars and a snively cold. We are to meet in two days for the final treatment to rid me of any lingering evil left by my malignant malady, and it had just better cure this cold as well."

Meanwhile Laura was typing away and I was between apricot-pit cures and an article on somebody in Switzerland who had a mysterious medicine that could only be had by going to his clinic and taking the treatment there. He didn't want "organized medicine" to steal his secret since they had been so scornful and disbelieving of his claims.

At our next early-morning rendezvous in the cafeteria, we had to pull over another table to make room for the eager ears waiting to hear Mary's latest. This embarrassed her. She didn't like being the center of attention. With goading, however, she cupped her hands around her cup, lowered her gaze into her coffee, and reported on her latest exploit.

"This was," she told us, "the very antithesis of the Chinese herbalist. A posh waiting room, all chrome and reflecting embossed wallpaper, stark black and white. Elegant receptionist. The plaque on the door had so many letters after the name I couldn't tell what it all meant. The receptionist informed me, in a rather kindly and patronizing fashion, that the clinician, whom she carefully refrained from calling doctor, had been trained in Mexico in the arts of ancient Mayan and Aztec natural healing. I expressed surprise, saying that I understood the Aztecs had been more apt to take a life than to save it. Her patter was so ingrained that she didn't even register my comment but went on to dwell on the "clinician's" European training in the use of electricity.

"After waiting a suitable time, I was shown into the inner sanctum—an office with all sorts of framed certificates on the wall, most having to do with service clubs, as nearly as I could tell at a glance. The great man himself was all porcelain-capped teeth, musky aftershave, and heavily pomaded hair, most artfully arranged. His stiffly starched white clinic coat had a stethoscope (which he never offered to use) hanging out of the pocket. He kept patting my hand, calling me 'my dear,' and saying, 'How awful' and 'Too, too dreadful,' as I gave him some symptoms pointing to a gastric malignancy. It did seem a stomach problem would overcome me if I stayed there very long. He also gave me a very verbose and meaningless harangue about electricity orienting molecules of health in one direction and disease in another. Then he hooked me up to a machine for all the world like a jukebox or pinball machine—all flashing lights with some bells and gurglings. It gave me a mild electric shock like the sort of things kids get at a fair for kicks. He pointed out to me that the chair on which I sat was oriented very carefully with a line on the floor which, he was pleased to say, had been placed there under direction of a true marine compass. Then there were three capsules to take, one every eight hours, and I was given an appointment to come back in a few days for follow-up treatment. The capsules were five dollars apiece and the consultation fee twelve. Back in my lab, I analyzed the material in the capsules. It was a mixture of cornstarch and salt."

We didn't see Mary over the Thanksgiving holiday, but the first day after vacation we met once more. She was weary, pale, and dispirited and announced sadly that she just couldn't keep up the remainder of her end of our bargain.

"Why ever not?" asked Laura, shocked at the idea. "You're doing such a splendid job. Our grade is really going to rest on your efforts. Ours are really only peripheral."

"It doesn't matter how they start out," Mary explained. "It all comes down, literally and figuratively, to the same thing in the end." Her voice took on an unwontedly indignant tone. "And it's my end at that. I've been back to that praying charlatan and that horribly perfumed 'clinician,' but I cannot go back to that Chinese herbalist. A coffee one is one thing and a tea and soapsuds one is another, but I cannot possibly permit that Chinaman to give me a ginseng high-colonic flush."

The Appointment

When you expect an appointment for residency training, know there is a vacancy, and know you are qualified, the angst really builds up when day after day and finally week after week passes and there is no letter in the mailbox.

Armando and I each needed either a year of a basic medical science, such as anatomy, physiology, or pathology, or a year in research for our general surgery training. We had decided that pathology would be most useful so had applied to hospitals in the Midwest that were associated with a medical school. Armando, not yet a United States citizen and therefore not qualified for the Veterans' Hospital, was appointed to the hospital next to the medical school. The stipend was to be thirty-five dollars per month. I applied to the Veterans' Hospital, where the pay was a glorious forty-five dollars a month. Now, from the relative comfort of retirement, the weird and wonderful ways in which the government can waste our money seems ludicrous. Then, when we were literally down to our last nickel, we were unable to see much mirth in the situation at all when the confirmation of my appointment failed to arrive.

It was Lucho, Armando's youngest brother, who finally told us why the six-week delay in the appointment and a cloak-and-dagger farce it was.

Lucho was middle management for one of the Columbian airlines. On a certain day, which we later realized was shortly after my application for a post as resident in pathology had been received, he was approached by Lydia, a stewardess, with a curious bit of news.

There had been, she said, a gentleman on a flight to Bogotá, who had consumed somewhat more than his fair share of the liquor on board and who had become, as a result, a bit talkative and confiding.

Lucho's dark eyes reflected his amusement as he told us he could understand the man's urge well enough as Lydia was unusually attractive—very curvaceous, great dark, soulful eyes, and all attentiveness.

The passenger told her, "in confidence of course, my dear," that he was being sent by the U.S. government (the CIA she thought he'd said) to do a very delicate investigation into the political leaning of a certain well-known family in Bogotá. The wife of one of the family members was being considered for a very sensitive position, and it was this gentleman's sole judgment that would assure the powers that be that such an appointment would not jeopardize the national security of the United States.

The stewardess, recognizing Lucho's family name, which happened to be a very unusual one, flattered the man as much as she could without being fatuous, but that seemed to be all the information she was able to unearth.

Lydia was as interested in impressing Lucho (whose position in the company was considerably senior to hers) as the CIA man had been in impressing her. More than that, Lucho was a very nice-looking man, not overly tall, but with an appealing personality and a robust sense of humor.

We wondered later if the government functionary had encountered Lydia on his return trip from Bogotá and, if so, what he might have said to her. Did he admit that Doña Eladia had been in her crypt for some years? That Don Carlos was somewhere between the bizarre and the incompetent in his senility? Did he tell her that the other members of the family were naturalized citizens of the United States, living politically dull lives in Miami?

And what of the appointment when it finally materialized? With whom was I to be consorting and communing daily that deep secrets exposed could be used to decimate the security of my country and lead to its utter downfall?

All day and every day I spent doing autopsies.

Nipples

Maternity and postpartum care were out of the Middle Ages by the time of the Second World War but only just. At least that's the way it was at Saint Margaret's Hospital.

With our maternity beds overflowing with servicemen's and warworkers' wives, we were still turning the patients over in bed for the first week of their two-week hospital stay. We gave them bed baths daily, castor oil and orange juice periodically, and enemas every third day. The only activity they managed for themselves, as nearly as we could tell, was to open their mouths—to eat, to demand service, or to complain.

With this lack of activity it was no wonder that the incidence of "milk leg," or clot formation in the deep veins of the calf, was fairly common. It led occasionally to an embolus or clot from one of these veins, which if it floated off into the lungs, could kill the patient suddenly, orphaning the newborn.

On the same level of patient management (and this was the standard of care throughout the country) was the preparation of baby formula. Mothers were not encouraged to nurse their infants, and few did. It was considered atavistic if not downright disgusting, not to mention inconvenient. Breasts were an item of personal decor and not functional in an intergenerational sense.

Various formulae were made up in the serving kitchen on the maternity floor, each physician favoring his own ingredients and proportions. Some were based on cows' milk, some on tinned milk, many had sugar, some had honey or corn syrup, etc.

The bottles had to be cleaned immediately after each feeding for they were old narrow-necked ones, and if the formula once dried the least little bit, it couldn't be removed. That was a catastrophe. Baby bottles were in increasingly short supply as the war years wore on.

Even more critical was the matter of the nipples. They were sterilized separately from the bottles, which were simply boiled in a huge pan. The nipples were done in a double boiler-steamer sort of affair to minimize the limpness that overcame them all too soon, thereby allowing the milk to flow all too freely and practically choke the poor babies.

Each of us coped with these problems in our own way. Magda went to bed the moment she got off duty and stayed curled up in a fetal ball until she had to get up for class. Looking back, she was in the throes of a deep depression. Evelyn became surly, and we all avoided her. Lacking an audience for her complaints, she just became more sour—angry because other people wouldn't wear her hair shirt. Melba retained her sweet good humor, worked harder, and acquired a Finnish boyfriend, whose mother plied her with the pastries that kept up her weight, strength, and good temper. And I, when I saw a patient turning herself over in bed, I turned a blind eye. Medical knowledge was one thing, but common sense was another. The patients had more and better food than we did and did nothing with their energy—not even producing milk. They were put in tight breast binders and put on stilbestrol to put an end to that foolishness. As a result of my sloth, if you will, no patient of mine ever had "milk leg."

Frances didn't change much under pressure. Under ordinary circumstances her movements and tongue were streets ahead of her thoughts, and now they were barely in the same time zone.

On this particular day, Ann, one of the senior nurses, was in the nursery alone, caring for half again as many babies as would be ideal. She had brought the babies back from their mothers, who had given them their two o'clock bottles; then she'd changed and reswaddled them before placing them in their basinets in front of the viewing window.

Ann raised the curtain so that the visitors could stand outside in the hall and make inane comments about the infants, who were so well wrapped that they all looked alike.

Rushing to the service kitchen at the other end of the hall with the bottles and nipples, Ann cleaned them as rapidly as possible and put them on the stove to sterilize. In her haste to get back to the nursery to bag up the soiled laundry, she somehow didn't get any or at least not enough water in the bottom of the double boiler.

Frances and I were doing our charting when a sudden wave of acrid fumes reached us. She was closest so she ran to the little kitchen. Her temperament hadn't deserted her even under stress. Instead of slamming the door shut and taking the pan from the stove, she jumped out of the door to the kitchen, stood in the middle of the corridor, and screamed down its length, to my amazement and the utter horror of the visitors, "Help! Annie! Your nipples are burning!"

Mistaken Identity

During the first years of my surgical practice, I volunteered one day a week at the tumor clinic. It served several counties, and as a result we saw a number of migrant workers from the mucklands of the state near Lake Okeechobee.

Rigoberto Vasquez was a Mexican migrant. He wasn't a migrant worker—just a migrant. The year before, somewhere between the cantaloupe of the Rio Grande valley, the bean-fields of Florida, and the strawberries of Pennsylvania, his brain had petered out.

With the stoic fatalism of the Mexican Indians, his family accepted his condition and with it the necessity to leave the children too young to work in the fields with him during the day. The lack of alternative equated acceptance with apathy. The grizzle-haired bronze-faced man wandered about the labor camp from day to day in a confused fashion, sometimes not completely clothed.

When the Public Health nurse made her rounds in the migrant camp and saw Rigoberto, she told his family that he must be taken to the tumor clinic to have the mass on his nose treated. The family took this news with passivity and resignation.

Surely, after all, it was *segun el Dios,* according to God.

All of this we heard from the nurse who brought him to the clinic. We examined him there and found the tumor to be cancerous and quite extensive. Since the bean season was nearly over and the family about to leave, the surgery needed to be done at once, hopefully in a one-stage procedure. With luck it could be done in such a manner that the patient could not easily pick it apart.

Admissions finally scratched up a bed in a two-bed room, into which another hapless male soul had already been admitted. The room was on the women's surgical wing, but perhaps on the following day there would be available beds on the men's wing to which they could be transferred.

That evening my new (and happily, bilingual) associate went to take a medical history and do a physical examination on the patient. The three-to-eleven nurse reported that Rigoberto didn't seem to be able to give a very coherent history but was obviously mightily impressed by this young man in his crisp white coat and the extremely detailed physical exam. Discussing it later, my associate remarked that he had failed to find any local evidence on Rigoberto's personal equipment that would give evidence of the primary infection of syphilis. In the light of his mental condition, tertiary syphilis had seemed a likely diagnosis and it would possibly have made some of the care more complicated.

Making early rounds the next morning to review lab tests before surgery, I arrived on second main to face an enraged charge nurse. Usually she was so calm and controlled, but now Mrs. Cohen's penetrating voice hit me head-on when I was still halfway down the corridor. "Doctor," she screeched, "you simply have to do something about that awful man. We just can't have him on this floor." She became almost incoherent as she continued charting temperatures at a furious rate, stabbing the graphic sheets angrily with her pen.

Rigoberto had seemed harmless enough to me in the tumor clinic, so I asked, "Why? What's he doing now?"

"Nothing at the minute. Father Fagan is in there trying to keep him in bed and in his room until time for his presurgical medication."

"Father Fagan?"

Mrs. Cohen's shoulders slumped against what had been a crisply starched uniform. "Yes. When he came at 5:00 A.M. to give last rites to the patient at the end of the hall everything was in a shambles and nothing was ready for him. He came back as soon as he finished passing communion on the other floors and is trying to help. I always knew these priests must be good for something practical, and even his few words of Spanish and his clerical collar have calmed the patient a bit, but we're still over an hour behind in our work."

"Well then, what was Señor Vasquez doing before?"

"What wasn't he doing?" Mrs. Cohen shrilled, tense again. "He's been up and down the hall all night, trying to jump into bed with the women patients. They've been hysterical, sitting on their call bells, the gatrectomy patient vomiting with fright. One poor soul, wakened out of a sound sleep, ran out onto the fire escape to shriek and woke up the patients on the floor above. Mr. Vasquez tripped over Mrs. Owen's tubing, knocked the weights around on Mrs. Varden's traction, and bumped into Miss Forsyth so hard as she came out of one of the rooms that the bedpan and emesis basin were sent flying out of her hands and went slopping and clattering down the hall floor." Mrs. Cohen's voice rose higher. "We can't have him, I tell you."

As I turned to go down the hall, Miss Forsyth and her medication cart flew by, rattling along well above the speed limit on a city street. Strands of hair straggled across her face, and her uniform was splotched with evil-looking stains.

A few minutes' talk in Spanish with Rigoberto solved the problem. I thanked Father Fagan and left him to his baby-sitting. That left me with the problem of how to tell Mrs. Cohen what Señor Vasquez had said.

Overburdened, understaffed, and with a patient dying (they are always at the far end of the hall), with no end in sight to the night's work or problems, I knew that some instant emotional relief would be the best thing to offer the exhausted nurses.

"And what *are* you going to do with that despicable man?" Mrs. Cohen's tones were insistent and shrill. "His behavior is . . . is . . . is impossible."

"Nothing," I replied.

"Nothing?" she screeched.

"No. If you just accept his basic premise, his behavior is not only understandable but quite, well, suitable."

"*Suitable!*"

"Yes. He thinks my associate, with his starched white jacket and consuming and detailed interest in private sexual apparatus, is the attendant in a high-class whorehouse."

Elegant Dining

Before being joined in practice by Armando, my husband, I was on emergency-room call for plastic surgery cases at two different hospitals twenty-four hours every day.

After some months of this, it seemed to me I was losing my perspective. A single stitch with a minute infection began to look as grievous as a face torn to fragments by a windshield.

With the way in which plastic surgery overlapped other specialties, it was necessary to secure the commitment of three other physicians. These indulgent gentlemen consisted of a general surgeon, an orthopedist, and an oral surgeon.

Next, a careful scrutiny of my pocketbook and an interview with a nearby travel agent led me to a modest hotel in Nassau for a four-day respite.

My room was comfortable though not luxurious. It looked out on the pool rather than the ocean—another concession to cost. That was not important since most of the time I spent outdoors anyway. With me were a number of books and my sketching pads. Each day was similar: an early swim in the ocean before the sun was too much for my fair skin, then a breakfast of fruit, quickbread, and coffee in the coffee shop; the remainder of the day was spent moving around in the shade of a large hibiscus bush next to the pool. From that location I could surreptitiously sketch some of the amazing bits of anatomy that were being flaunted by the pool and do it under the camouflage of my books.

A snack of tropical fruit from the market midday then an

early afternoon nap prepared me for the remainder of the day under the hibiscus bush. A dusk swim and a simple meal in the coffee shop again were followed by a long evening walk along the beach and made for a great night's sleep.

I was much refreshed after three days of this, so on the fourth and last day I consulted my purse again and decided I could afford to splurge and have dinner in the main dining room.

After a refreshing shower, I dressed carefully in a simple but rather nice green and white pique dress that I had made just for times like this. White sandals and a small white envelope purse completed my outfit, and as I waited to be seated in the dining room, the mirrors by the entry told me that I'd be no disgrace to the establishment.

The maître d' seated me at a pleasant little table overlooking the pool area and, beyond it, the ocean. Presently, after I'd scrutinized the menu, the waiter arrived. He was very tall, very black, and moved with a fluid effortless grace to take the menu from me and unfold the napkin to place it in my lap. As he bent down and inclined his head toward me, his dark eyes flashed with vitality as we discussed the meal.

"And has madame decided upon the entree?"

"Yes, may I please have the Cornish game hen?"

A shining smile rewarded me as he approved my choice and wrote it on his order pad. "You will find it most excellent. And would madame care for conch chowder or a clear soup?"

We discussed that for a few moments. His interest in describing the precise local seasonings in the chowder was as intense as his effort to ply his pen and put the exact request in writing.

The chowder was served with a flourish, followed in a minute or so with a question. "And is the flavor to madame's taste?" Assured that it was, his step was exceptionally buoyant as he retired temporarily to the kitchen.

After removing my soup bowl, the waiter returned, favored me with a beaming smile, and embarked upon matters of extreme importance: the salad dressing and a vegetable to complement the entree.

The tamarind viniagrette and the peas in mint sauce selected, he bent his head once again over the leather-covered order pad and wrote industriously. The serious attentiveness was relieved by a delightfully spontaneous expression of approval and his dark eyes glistened with pleasure when his recommendations were accepted.

"With the selections madame has chosen, would not a light sweet, for instance a mango sorbet to accompany her coffee, give madame pleasure?" Once again the pen moved rapidly to record the item.

The entire dinner was served most deftly and solicitiously. I felt my final splurge, while self-indulgent, was well worth the inroads it had made on the vacation budget.

"It has been," my waiter intoned, "a great pleasure to serve madame." A semibow and his charming smile accompanied the placement of the bill face down on my table.

Thanking him profusely as he drew out my chair for my departure, I picked up the bill with my purse and, after leaving a rather nice tip, took it to the cashier's desk. While waiting my turn there, a niggling thought came to me that my delightful mentor's writing must be very crabbed and cramped to fit on the small slip of paper. It would have to be writing totally at odds with his otherwise loose, graceful, fluid motions.

Curious, I idly flipped the bill over to read on the front portion the entire gamut of intricate reminders. There, inscribed in large block letters, was one terse word—HEN.

Organics

Trying to be an organic gardener when you lack animals of your own and have no horsey friends from whom to panhandle by-products isn't easy.

Nonetheless, on the double lot on the west side of the intracoastal waterway, I'd managed to grow coconuts, loquats, peanuts, papayas, carissas, pineapples, Surinam cherries, carambolas, mabolos, kumquats, grumichamas, and roseapples, in addition to several varieties of bananas and citrus.

Armando, my husband, enjoyed looking at the flowers and making daiquiris from the fresh fruit, but his interest wasn't sustained enough to learn the names of many of the trees and plants. This embarrassed him mildly when people would stop by when I wasn't home and ask what this tree or that potted plant might be. He finally solved this by going around and, as I told him what they were, writing the names on the tree bark or on the pots. Unfortunately, he used indelible ink and couldn't understand why some fairly knowledgeable folks gave him peculiar looks about some of the potted plants. They had grown large and potbound, so I'd repotted the begonias into a larger pot labeled maiden hair fern, etc.

We'd been having rather a lot of rain, which had washed the fertilizer right on down through the sand and left the fruit trees high and dry for food. As a matter of fact, a seventeen-inch rainfall sent our seawall to sea and left an Olympic-pool-sized portion of the lake where the lawn had been—between the house and the sea wall.

Arrangements for the repair of the seawall and sprinkler system had been made (by myself of course). Armando's contribution had been a shrug of the shoulders and one of his usual mumbled mixed metaphors, "Out of the frying pan into the bushes."

I was determined to have him shoulder his share of the responsibility, so when an ad appeared in the Sunday paper that a nearby supply store had a sale on composted cow manure at seventy-seven cents a bag, the opportunity was welcome.

Exaggerating his limp, drooping his shoulders more than usual, and cultivating a beleaguered look in his dark eyes, Armando went to the garage for the station wagon. As he opened its door, he turned his head back to inquire, "How many bags?"

"Ten," I answered. Who knew when a sale like this would come again and it would be possible to corral him into helping?

Forty minutes later, I was cleaning the sprinkler heads when the station wagon turned into the drive. I went to unload the bags, since it was a total misery for his multiple-operated-on back to even try. The station wagon was empty, and when Armando opened its door and got out, it was apparent by the downward slope of the outer ends of his eyebrows that something had completely flummoxed, baffled, and perplexed him. It had been a long time since I'd seen him with such an expression of incredulous incomprehension.

"So what happened?" I asked.

"*Pues, entonces*" (well, then), he replied, "I said to the checkout girl, 'May I please pay for ten bags of the composted cow manure, and I'll drive around back where they can load it up for me?' She was one of those brightly cheerful young

41

things and looked the soul of distress when she said, 'I'm so sorry, sir, we are out of that item.' When I sort of asked, 'Oh?' her expression was one of uncertainty; then she gave me a smile of delight as she suddenly thought of the perfect excuse and burbled on, 'You see, the machine that makes it broke down!' "

Opportunity

No one attracts my admiration as much as the person who can turn a devastating or bizarre event into a stupendous success, in short, a first-class opportunist.

On a small scale this happened at the same time that the seventeen-inch rainfall took our seawall to sea; the summer of 1972, I seem to recall.

Florida, at least in its southern portions, is really just one gigantic sand spit, with little to no gradient for drainage. This, of course, was the basis for the Everglades, that river of grass that seasonally was a great sheet of water just a few inches deep, that moves imperceptibly slowly through the native saw grass toward the Gulf of Mexico. That is, it did until we messed it up with dikes and drainage and "improvements," which have been a disaster nearly destroying a unique ecosystem.

The hospital in question was in a portion of the area that was flat, flat, flat. It had been a cowpasture, and in its early days, the hospital's first-floor patients were occasionally startled by the sight of an inquiring, cud-chewing bovine face poked in between the window louvers.

I had mixed feelings about the physical plant of the hospital. It had obviously been planned without reference to some rather basic sanitation considerations. For instance, the newborns had to be carried through the waiting area for emergency-room patients on the way to the newborn nursery. Think of all the colds, flu, and other things there that one shouldn't have to be exposed to during the first hour of life.

Then there were the carpets. In my opinion, they were not cleanable in the sanitary sense that should apply to hospitals. In addition to embedded dirt, the odd bits of emesis and other personal effluvia embedded there would make a cockroach queasy.

The building itself, though, was built around an open courtyard that was of modest size but which gave a pleasant added light to the surrounding rooms. It also was a warm, sunny spot on cool days for ambulatory and wheelchair patients and staff. Likewise, there was shade under its two trees when the sun was too aggressive, altogether an agreeable feature in a hospital.

But then the rain came, and the hospital administrator (who was at home wrestling with a swale, driveway and garage under half a foot of water) was startled by a call from the nursing supervisor announcing that water was a foot and a half deep in the patio and rising rapidly.

Mr. Revers rushed to the hospital and through the carpeted corridors to the patio door, under which the determined water was already making its single-minded way, discoloring the rug as it went. Whether he shared my opinion of carpeted hospitals or not, I don't know, but he looked suspiciously smug when he told me about it later. Mr. Revers told me that he said to the nursing supervisor, "I must check the drainage from the patio." With this announcement he opened the door to step into the patio, and as he did, a tidal wave of water nearly swept him off his feet. It rushed on down the hall, pushing small bits of flotsam, leaves, etc., from the patio on its leading edge. It didn't take a genius to see that the carpets were forever ruined.

In my heart of hearts I can't help wondering—did he not know there was no drainage from the patio? As might have been anticipated, the insurance company felt lucky and was considerably relieved when it was decided to use vinyl flooring instead of recarpeting. I seem to remember that he even persuaded them to lower the insurance premiums and provide a sort of sump pump for the patio so that such an expensive problem could not arise there again.

The Inquisition

Most elderly people accept life's uncertainties with a certain amount of equanimity; either that or over time they have learned to control their facial expressions so that their true feelings are masked a bit. Theodore Clinger was a radical exception. The first time he came to the office, his pupils were dilated with fright, and had it been a second-story office, I'd have stood between him and the window—just in case. Almost as startling as his appearance of absolute terror was the aspect of his dentition. Never had I, in all my born days, seen such a jumble of teeth. They were so higgledy-piggledy that it was almost impossible to tell which were upper teeth and which were from the lower jaw.

Dr. Potter had, of course, called about the referral of the elderly widower and warned me. Apparently, Mr. Clinger's wife had expired in a northern hospital after a particularly difficult, gruesome, painful, sad, and prolonged illness. When Doctor Potter had first seen the small skin cancer on Mr. Clinger's ear and suggested that it be surgically removed, the patient had reacted with utter panic. Dr. Potter said that he'd thought Mr. Clinger might have a stroke right then and there so the patient was sedated for a bit then Dr. Potter suggested that perhaps they might try radiation therapy. Mr. Clinger wasn't happy about that either since the radiotherapy would be done in a hospital, but he calmed down fairly well when it was explained that he just had to go there for a few visits for a short while at a time.

It's a bit difficult to say why the tumor didn't respond to the therapy, but it was probably because of the contour of the ear and the problem of delivering an equal dose to both sides of the fold, as it were. These things are so much better now with the new machines and techniques, but in any case, Dr. Potter had finally persuaded him to come over to our office, saying that he knew we had a small operating room there and perhaps we could do something for him without hospitalization.

I spent a good bit of time with him in the consulting office then asked him to step into the examining room and sit on the edge of the table. His eyes darted furtively toward the door, and he stammered, "I don't have to lie down?"

"No, I can really beam this examining lamp very easily, and then I won't have to bend over. It will be easier for both of us." With that he finally managed a phantom of a smile . . . and there was the startling mouth of teeth again. It brought to mind a picture of a jumbled heap of bones, potsherds, and teeth I'd seen in an artcle about an excavation of prehistoric animals and broken pots—the ultimate jigsaw puzzle.

Dragging my mind back to the patient's problem, I examined the ear carefully. It seemed best to postpone peering about for similar lesions until he was more at ease. In fair skins these things do have a tremendous tendency to be multiple after a certain age, and he appeared about seventy-four. The lump was only about a centimeter and a half in diameter, and fortunately, surgically it was located over a portion of the cartilage that bulged outward. This meant there was a valley on the reverse side of the ear where skin for repair could be readily mobilized.

Back in the consulting office, Mr. Clinger appeared a little less frantic.

"It is my custom to give a bit of a sedative in advance, even for patients who have relatively small problems," I explained.

"Do you have a friend who could drive you and wait for you while we get rid of this little affair?" The use of the words *sedative, small,* and *little* seemed to put the poor fellow more at ease. "This won't bother you any more than a trip to the dentist."

This time the smile was a little easier. "To be honest," he said sheepishly, "I've never had to go to the dentist. I originally came from a small hamlet in Texas—just a crossroads, really. No one there ever had tooth decay. Something in the water they said. Since there were no dentists, there were no ortho-dontists within a hundred miles—if that—and in any case, doing something about my teeth wasn't something my folks would have been concerned about. They were too busy trying to keep food on the table with the erratic weather in that dry, dusty, tornado-prone land."

I nodded my head. "This I understand very well. I grew up in the dust bowl, in Dakota. It probably wasn't much better during those years, though usually there were crops to a greater or lesser degree in our territory."

Now that he had control of himself, he drew his slightly portly five and a half feet of height up in the chair and announced fairly firmly, "About transportation here, that won't be a problem. I have a friend who is also retired. What day will this be?"

We agreed on the following Tuesday at 8:00 A.M. He was to skip breakfast and take his sedative at a quarter of seven. That would give it plenty of time to work, even if his stomach was upset at the prospect ahead of him.

Came the following Tuesday and he lurched in on the arm of another gentleman of about the same age. "I feel drunk and foolish. Maybe I'd better lie down."

We herded him into the small surgery and tried to make him comfortable on his side.

"Now, Mr. Clinger, as we go along, I'll tell you just what

to expect so neither of us will get upsetting surprises. First, my nurse will scrub your ear and the area around it with a special solution to clear away any surface germs."

He giggled. "It's been close to seventy years since anyone has had to scrub my ears for me. Mother had a vicious hand with a washcloth, I tell you. Said if I wouldn't do a good job, she'd really show me how."

"I'm afraid my mother shared the same horrible attitude. Now, the next thing we do is to place a sterile piece of cloth with a hole for your ear over this area. There now, can you peer out from under it?"

"Yes, but the view of the blank wall isn't inspiring."

"Sorry about that, Mr. Clinger, but the dancing girls don't come to work this early. I'm going to pinch the skin of your ear now so that I can see just where this might be attached to the cartilage."

While I was pinching his ear, a fine thirty-gauge needle was slipped in under my fingers and a small bit of local anesthetic injected. By doing this very slowly, he wasn't aware of what was happening. Warning him about another pinch, I pushed the needle through the cartilage and numbed the back of the ear as well. The nurse then removed the sterile towel that had covered the instrument tray and slid it in from the adjacent room. We had felt that the premature sight of even a covered Mayo stand might cause the patient to flee precipitously.

The actual excision of the lesion was only the work of a few seconds. It was placed on a gauze sponge and dropped into the hands of the nurse, who had a specimen bottle already labeled for it.

"Now, you will feel that I am bending your ear back and forth, sir, because we must close the little place where your tumor was."

"Do you mean it is already gone?"

"Yes, but like so many things in life, tearing something down takes much less time than building it up. I have to borrow a little tongue of skin from the back of your ear where you won't miss it and draw it through to close the space that is not covered now. You will hear a little buzz from the machine that stops the bit of ooze." It had seemed prudent not to refer to the surgical defect as a raw area.

After about fifteen minutes, during which time it seemed that the patient might have dozed a little, I warned him, "Now you will feel a little tugging as this is being stitched together. After that we will put quite a large bandage on your ear so that if you roll over on it during the night when you are asleep, no harm will be done to the healing process."

The nurse had placed the proper bandages on the sterile table for me and poured a few drops of sterile mineral oil on a gauze sponge. Placing it right over the wound would allow any few drops of ooze to go through it to the dry dressing and would prevent crusts from sticking to the bandage. That way, when the dressing was removed, the early healing wouldn't be disturbed.

After the bulky bandage was in place, we mobilized the patient, who was now more or less sober. In the mirror of my consulting office he looked at himself and remarked, "It looks as if I might have lost the battle."

"That's right, Mr. Clinger. Just don't tell anyone that the winner was a young woman."

Over the next couple of follow-up visits, we got to know each other quite well. While doing his dressing, we discussed our gardens and his painting, a hobby he had developed after moving to the area. Often he would bring roses from his garden or root a cutting of one of his favorite plants for me. He may not have enjoyed coming to the office, but it seemed to hold no fear for him anymore.

We hadn't seen him for several months after the ear was healed, when he phoned one day.

"I think I've grown another one of these pesky tumors. This time it's on my cheek, and it seemed more sensible to call you directly than to bother Dr. Potter with it. Was that all right?"

Reassured that we would be happy to see him, an appointment was made. Sure enough, it was another skin cancer. This time all went very easily, and when he returned to have his sutures removed, he could hardly wait to tell me the latest in his life.

"The other day I was out pruning the bushes," he began. "I looked up to see this female person bearing down on me, coming over the grass from the sidewalk; you know, the kind of woman who goes through life using her chin and her bosoms to elbow everyone out of her way? Well, this was the prototype of aggressive females. She started out by demanding to know if I owned this property. It's a retirement cottage on a midsized lot, as I've told you. Her attitude irritated me, but curiosity led me to go along with the conversation just to see how outrageous it might become, so I admitted that I owned the place."

Next, she said, "Do you live alone?"

"Yes, madam," I told her.

"Do you do all of your own garden work?"

"Oh, yes." By this time I was mightily irritated.

Another insistent question. "Do you cook for yourself?"

"Every meal," I told her.

With this, she stepped right up close in front of me, shoved her face into mine, and brusquely asked, "Are those your own teeth?"

Brassieres

A glance at her chart didn't prepare me for the new patient's aggressive attitude. Her name, according to the chart, was Mrs. Kelandon, and she was a widow from Night Heron Hideaway, a very exclusive golf and country club community some few miles to the north of the office.

Mrs. Kelandon wasted no time on the amenities, nor did she give me an opportunity to inquire what I might do for her. She stalked into the office, skewered me on an imperious stare, as she looked down at me—and I'm fairly tall—, jabbed her finger at my chest, and rasped out her order. "Look here, you, I want you to cut these goddamn things off." With that order, she slammed the sides of her bosoms with her hands. The bosoms didn't bang together. They couldn't for they were far too tightly encased in what must have been the most substantial brassiere of all time. A memory and a vivid mental image materialized of the webbing on the threshing machines that were in use on the grain-growing prairies during my childhood.

Startled and bemused, I indicated a chair across from my desk and there she sat, stiff and upright.

"Why, after seventy-eight years of your life, do you suddenly find this problem insupportable?" I inquired.

"I'll have you know," she announced decisively, "that I play at least eighteen holes of golf every day and walk all of it. Up north in the summer, it's the same, except that the course there is in the foothills and the walking is up and down." She looked distastefully at the front of her dress, raised her gravelly voice in outrage, and complained, "The goddamn things get in the way of my golf swing."

It wasn't hard to be sympathetic. I didn't have the problem myself, but the first two patients who had been sent to me for reduction mammaplasty had corroborated my notion that too much was more of a problem than too little where breasts were concerned.

One of those first patients had been sent by a pulmonary specialist. Her lungs couldn't expand properly against the burden of enormous and weighty breasts. The second had come from an orthopedist, whose prescription of a shoulder brace for a patient with severe neck and shoulder pain had proven ineffective in the face of huge, heavy bosoms. Even among my friends, I had seen chronic ulceration under the breasts and severe grooving of the soft tissue over a clavicle deformed by the constant pressure of bra straps.

Mrs. Kelandon may have been seventy-eight years old, but in my mind, that was a relative matter. Anyone who walked at least eighteen holes a day and played a vigorous game of golf could certainly recline quietly under anesthesia on an operating table for the hours it took to remove most of the offending mass and reshape the breast mounds bilaterally. Positioning and replacing the nipples was fiddly and time consuming but certainly not very traumatic.

The patient showed relatively little interest in the details of the procedure—where the scars would be, how long it would take them to fade, the length of time for follow-up care, etc. Her only comments after my explanations were, "I don't care if I'm flat as a new bride's biscuit, and whether I have any nipples or not is of no concern. What would I use them for anyway? What I want to know is how much of all this can you get rid of for me and how soon can I play golf again?"

Privately I felt that reducing her breasts below a C cup

would make the proportions of her height, hips, and shoulders a clothing problem so I settled on that for a goal, thinking that the startling volume reduction would make her feel quite flat.

All went well with surgery and healing as Mrs. Kelandon was indeed in fit condition. A couple of months later, at the end of her follow-up period, Mrs. Kelandon arrived in the office looking so smug that I couldn't restrain a comment.

"You look very pleased with yourself—like the canary that went out and ate up the pussycat. Did you make a hole in one?"

"No, nothing like that, but you know I should have given those custom-made bras of mine to my cook. She's a very nice black lady, unfortunately, built just like I was. Trouble is, I didn't really want her to know what I'd done so this morning, as it was her day off, I went down to the secluded lower corner of the garden and had a bra-burning party for myself. Do you know," and with this she gave me a conspiratorial grin, "that I don't even have to wear a bra to play golf now if I don't want to?"

A Noble Calling

Before it became a prejorative word, I'd have said that social workers were a *queer* lot. Some can be so inventive and ingenious in the ways they devise to accomplish the impossible, but another group seem to have entered the field just to wallow in other people's emotional garbage. Then there are those who, depending on one's vintage, are thought of as "not quite with it," "out to lunch," or "off the wall."

Mrs. Lacey's wall was already listing and cracked. Bronx born and bred, she had sold herself to herself as an authentic if somewhat superannuated Southern Belle, replete with a bunch of false curls bobbing down the back of her neck à la Scarlett O'Hara. Her accent—when she didn't forget—was an affected mouthful of cotton "Suthun."

Mrs. Lacey's skirts had so much material in them that hoops could have been hidden underneath and never made a ripple. It was a credit to the innate cleverness of an illiterate Negro more than to her bald luck that Wahoo Washington would arrive within some tenuous connection to his appointed time at clinics, hospitals, or anywhere else. Today was surgery day, particularly rehabilitation, and I was the lucky plastic surgeon.

Somehow, together they had muddled their way to the clinic, and Wahoo's chart was in the box on the wall outside of the treatment room. It was meager. A piece of scrap paper clipped to the folder said "burn scars." Inside there was nothing. It didn't take a medical sleuth to know that some overburdened surgical resident in a teaching hospital hadn't gotten around to dictating a summary of several months' hospitalization. With every week that passed, the notations would be a murkier memory. I knew; I'd been there. Spying Mrs. Lacey sashaying down the dreary hall with her mincing steps, I escaped by entering the treatment room, where the patient sat on the edge of the examining table.

The direct sun boiling into the miniscule cubicle was blinding, but there was a fleeting image of a hideously gruesome jack-o-lantern on a black night. Eyes adjusting to the light, this resolved partially into a large black blob and, within the upper portion, three small white blobs. The large black mass was a severely deformed person and the two uppermost white blobs were the lower portions of the whites of his eyes, rolled to the uppermost extreme. The other white bit was an irregular line of teeth completely exposed by the pull of heavy scar that tethered his chin and lower lip tightly down to his chest wall.

Even a cursory look at Wahoo Washington would provide a good insight not only into his medical history but into the health of the district budget for the medically indigent.

Taut, shiny, heavy scarring fused the patient's arms to his chest wall. Even tighter scar tissue pulled his chin down onto his chest and his lower lip down so far that the red gums were exposed below the roots of his lower teeth. His shoulders were rolled forward and down, almost touching the sides of his face. All of the scars on the chest had a regular pattern of pebbling. That told me where he had been treated. There was a new gadget that made staggered slits in split-thickness skin grafts so that they could be pulled out and expanded like a mesh. The university hospital had one; and true, a little skin would go much farther, but the resulting scar, especially in black skin, gave this bumpy tire-tread look. The scar was at least as thick as a tire. Almost interminable physiotherapy probably could have prevented the adhesion between arms and chest, but once the raw areas were healed, the surgery residents had lost interest and the county wasn't about to pay the costs of endless physiotherpay for what was not a life-threatening condition.

So, Wahoo could barely feed himself, couldn't bathe himself, and was prone to lung infections because the scar was so constricting that his breathing was very shallow.

"Tell me, Mr. Washington," I asked (for I was a northerner and adults to me were Mister, regardless of color), "how did all this come about?"

"Well, ah'd had a few drinks and was a-smokin' in bed when it caught fire . . . ," his voice trailed off. He tried to smile, but the distorton of his mouth only intensified the grimace and pulled his lower lids down to expose more the lower whites of his eyes.

My mind ran over the possibilities. Ideally, of course, the neck should be released first so that an endotracheal tube could be used to administer anesthesia. No way could one be gotten into place with this acutely flexed neck. Further, digging a hole through that heavy scar using just local anesthesia would be a two-person job. The local anesthesia needles would bend or, worse, break off. Then there was the ogre of the budget. Once released and grafted, a padded heavy steel brace lined with goatskin would have to be custom made to keep Wahoo's neck from contracting down onto his chest again. These were very expensive, and there was no use expecting funding this close to the end of the fiscal year. And then there was the physiotherapy. Wahoo was from the Glades and would have to be domiciled at the county hospital (which, in reality, was not a hospital but sort of a custodial extended-care facility) while he had daily or twice-daily treatment for weeks. We'd have to go on a long waiting list for a bed there after he was discharged from the acute-care hospital. Where to start?

"Mr. Washington, I think we'd better release your right arm so that you can feed and take care of yourself better. With some sedative, I can do that and graft it, using just local anesthesia. We'll get on a waiting list for the county hospital, and that should come through shortly after my new associate arrives.

"All the other surgery, excepting your right arm, will take several operations and is a two-man job. After he comes, my associate will be captain of your ship and I'll help. He's better trained for this sort of thing than I am."

Wahoo nodded. He had been most of this route before and had a pretty good idea what was coming.

I told him about the neck brace and the airplane splints he would have to wear to keep his arms out at right angles from his body so they wouldn't fuse to his chest again. Together we looked ahead to the better part of a year of intermittent surgery, dressings, therapy, etc.

A ladylike tap at the door announced Mrs. Lacey. "Transport back to the Glades is in forty-five minutes, Doctor. Will my client be ready?" Mrs. Lacey was too genteel to call anyone Wahoo and obviously considered herself too much of a southern white lady to call him Mister.

"Yes, Mrs. Lacey," I assured her. "He will be with you in five minutes."

Turning to the patient again, I said, "This is a pretty drawn-out affair, as you know, Mr. Washington. How do you feel about that?" Cooperation could make or break these long-term things, and it didn't make sense to begin unless finishing were a realistic expectation.

"Ah jes' rolls wid dem punches, Doctah," was his reply. Life lay lightly on Wahoo's shoulders.

When the examining room door was opened for him to leave, Mrs. Lacey could be seen down at the end of the hall. She was making ineffectual fluttering motions with her hands and chattering animatedly at the poor secretary, distracting her from coping with the patients lined up on the benches before her.

Six months went by and finally Wahoo's neck and both arms were released. From some of the black ward attendants, we heard that he occasionally left the county hospital for the hospitality of the Blue Heron bar. Some of the buckles on his neck brace would be undone so it just flapped around, but when we saw him in clinic, things were generally progressing fairly well. We knew why the result on his right arm wasn't as good as the left. Wahoo couldn't drink very well with both arms up in airplane splints and he *was* right-handed.

A couple of years passed and Wahoo no longer needed to come to the clinic, but he came to my mind providentially one day. Mrs. Lacey was clattering down the dark hall toward me on her high heels, voluminous skirts twitching this way and that.

Fishing frantically around inside my head for a subject of conversation that would be self-limiting, I queried, "Mrs. Lacey, you remember Wahoo Washington, who was referred here by Rehabilitation? Just what was it we were rehabilitating him toward anyway?"

Mrs. Lacey turned sideways so she could posture, with her face looking archly back over her shoulder. "You didn't *know*, Doctor?" she twittered. Her heavily mascaraed lashes fluttered in their smudge, and her smile was coy as befits one who is the possessor of great knowledge about to be revealed in all its glory. Proudly she announced, "He was the bootlegger in Belle Glade."

Shana

Looking back through the retrospectoscope, Shana's injury was doubtless a matter of deliberate child abuse. We weren't tuned in to those things back then, and the idea that someone would deliberately injure their own child was unthinkable. As a result, the story her mother gave to explain the burn on Shana's face was accepted at face value. The burn on the cheek and ear were deep and the edges perfectly round. That there was no fuzziness of those edges and no burns from splashed boiling liquid should have been a clue that the hot pan had been applied forcefully and deliberately to Shana's face.

The little black toddler had been on the ward for several days when I was asked to see her. The general surgeon who had been called when she was brought to the emergency room had given the orders that kept her comfortable and the burn clean. The area was now ready for grafting, and he phoned to ask if I would take over the case since the problem was on her face.

The hospital was still a matter of segregated floors in those days, and the black pediatric ward was at the far end of a long hall. Mrs. Fountain was the head nurse there, a pudgy white lady somewhere between motherly and grandmotherly. Mrs. Fountain didn't deal in paper shuffling. She delegated that and spent all of her efforts caring for "her" children, both physically and emotionally. She loved all of "her" children, even the occasional unlovable one, and they blossomed under her care. As she worked she sang little songs that taught numbers and ABCs and, in Shana's case, her first few words.

Shana's mother didn't visit often. As far as I recall, she only came a few times before Shana's graft was healed. That was several weeks as the graft had to be a full-thickness one so that as she grew the corner of her eye wouldn't be distorted or her mouth drawn up on that side. The donor site where the full thickness of skin was removed had to be grafted in turn with split-thickness skin, the healing of which tended to be a bit slow in an infant not yet toilet trained. A urine poultice doesn't hasten healing.

All this while, other training went on apace. Mrs. Fountain taught Shana to say "Mama" against the day when her mother (in her cook's helper white uniform) might visit.

Finally, several days after her discharge from the hospital, Shana was brought to the office by her mother, who was in street clothes for the visit. Shana was first in the afternoon. We scheduled children that way so they wouldn't be irritable and fussy as they were apt to become if they had to wait their turn. At the same time, arriving a bit early for her appointment was "Mrs. Occidental Petroleum," who was to have sutures removed from an area on her face where a skin cancer had been removed.

Ever the gracious lady, "Mrs. Occidental Petroleum" spoke to Shana's mother to commiserate with her about the little girl's burn. The nurse was busy on the phone so I opened the waiting room door to call Shana and her mother into the dressing room. None of us were prepared for the result of Mrs. Fountain's careful teaching for Shana had learned to associate the word "Mama" with someone in white.

It took all the stamina of the patrician lady's poise and breeding to keep her face straight when the little black toddler spied my white clinic coat, held her arms out to me, and shrieked happily, "Mama."

61

Two-Way Street

As Armando once said, "One man's beast is another man's burden." For physicians, the telephone is both bane and blessing.

We once had to have our home phone number changed because the Harmony Hotel's number was only one digit different. It was on the other side of the tracks and catered to instant couples. Apparently there was also a sort of "take out" service for those who wanted their home comforts at home or were too far gone in their inebriation to make their way to that place of action.

It wasn't unusual when the phone rang at 1:00 A.M. or 2:00 A.M. or 3:00 A.M. for a muzzy voice to want to know, "Ish Gloria there?" When told no, they would say, "Well, maybe her name wassh Alish."

An internist of ours had a similar problem, but it was with a well-known pizza-peddling outfit. Wakened from a sound sleep by an impatient voice wanting to know how soon an extra large pizza with pepperoni and mushrooms could be delivered, she solved the problem to her immense satisfaction.

"What is the address?" she would ask. Then in a few moments, apparently after taking down the address, she would say, "You are in luck. We are having a special promotion and will be including six large Pepsis free of charge. If you like, for an extra seventy-five cents, you may have an extra four toppings, for instance, would you like olives, sausage, peppers, and anchovies?" After all of these pleasantries, she would roll over and fall sound asleep, contented with her night's effort.

Then there was the matter of the "peas in the night." One of our pediatrician friends had had a day such as one has occasionally—an overflowing office schedule to begin with and two emergency rooms to cover during the holiday and flu season. He himself was coming down with the bug and felt perfectly wretched. At 2:00 A.M. the phone woke him from a sleep that had finally been achieved by elevating his head and stuffing it with nose drops and cough drops.

The voice on the phone complained, "You know, I don't think that peas are agreeing with the baby."

"Who is this?" he asked.

"Betsy Norman's mother. Those peas just don't seem to sit well with her."

"Why do you think the peas are bothering her?" he wanted to know.

"Oh, I don't know. She just doesn't seem right somehow."

"Tell me, what she is doing now? What symptoms does she have of any trouble?"

A shocked voice answered. "Why, she's asleep now, of course."

Resignedly, our friend told the woman to discontinue the peas, but the thoughtless insensitivity, yes, the injustice of the encounter, rankled so that he couldn't get back to sleep. By the time a call came from the emergency room at 4:30 A.M., he was simply seething with resentment. Arriving at the hospital, sniffling and coughing, he whiled away a few minutes with the phone book while the nurses set up a suture tray.

Dialing the Norman residence, he heard a sleepy female voice on the line. "Hello," it said, "who is this?"

"It's your pediatrician. I called to find out if those were fresh peas or canned peas or frozen peas."

He was telling us about it later and said he was amazed

that as soon as he placed the phone back on its cradle, he noticed that his respiratory symptoms had largely, magically, vanished.

The Nugget

Psychiatry has always seemed to me to be too insubstantial and impalpable to class as a science, it's so full of abstractions as well as conflicting and constantly changing theories. Nonetheless, I remember with admiration a nurse instructress I had at the state mental hospital where I did my rotation as a student nurse.

From the Menninger Clinic in Kansas, she was very practical and full of good common sense. She taught us one thing that has gleamed through the years as a twenty-four-carat nugget. "Remember," she admonished, "even in the most bizarrely misconstrued observation or perverted misinterpretation, there is, at the bottom, some grain of truth. Sometimes, with patience at raveling out the twisted skeins of understanding, the perception of an event to a person you might consider insane is closer to the essence of the matter than your understanding of the situation." That bit of advice leapt into my head the moment I heard from sniggering evening nurses the story of Professor Gaynor's malady and the interpretation of the situation made by his nurse.

Mrs. Strom didn't know about this theory. She was the day-shift private-duty nurse caring for Professor Gaynor, who was better known for his alcoholic consumption than his professional abilities. Having retired to Palm Beach, he continued to dissipate his family inheritance on liquor and hospitalization for the ravages thereof. Truly his physicians had long since despaired of him, and each hospitalization was thought to be his last.

On this particular morning, Mrs. Strom scanned his chart, saw nothing unusual, and promptly at seven entered his room with a professionally cheery, "Good morning, Professor Gaynor. How is everything this morning?"

"As usual," he replied. Then, after a brief pause, he raised his eyebrows over his bloodshot, baggy eyes in a questioning manner and asked, "But have they caught that creature yet?"

"Caught what creature?" With this, Mrs. Strom's mind raced, and to herself she thought, *Oh, oh, here it is finally—the DTs.*

"I don't know for certain, but I believe the animal is called an anteater. It was scrabbling along the baseboards, sniffing. It had a rather long nose."

"If you'll excuse me, Professor, I'll go see what news there is of it before your breakfast arrives."

Her starched uniform rustled crisply as Mrs. Strom hastened to the chart desk, intending to phone the professor's doctor. *On second thought,* she mused, *why bother him? He needs his sleep if he's still in bed and there's nothing to do or order for the patient that hasn't already been done.* With that decision made, she simply noted the event on the chart and carried on with the day's work—breakfast, bathing the patient's bloated body, and keeping an ear cocked for further odd remarks.

A small item in the evening *Palm Beach Times* announced that the escaped pet of a couple of Texans living in a mobile home next to the hospital had been run to ground in the linen closet of the women's ward. According to the policeman who caught it, the animal was a harmless coatimundi.

One-Night Stand

Talk about Zorba the Greek! He wasn't a patch on my friend Nicholas Malavides. Nick doesn't only love life; he adores it, worships it, practically wallows in it. Nick is one of those intense citizens who invest 110 percent of their attention and energy into whatever engrosses them at the moment. He fairly thrums with his enthusiasms. Surgically, it's ears. Jug ears, shell ears, cup ears, plain lop ears, those that have chunks removed for tumor, bitten off for revenge or in passion—Nick devotes the attention to them that other men reserve for 38-24-34 blondes. When I saw him the other day, he had just finished giving a paper at one of the plastic surgeons' groups on yet another nifty and ingenious method of rectifying a bizarre problem with the ear cartilage.

Knowing that his second love was fishing, I spoke to him about it. "Nick, where have you been fishing lately?"

He tossed an unruly thatch of dark hair from his forehead, and his black eyes glittered with the memory. "Let me tell you about it. A really stupendous trip. We were staying in one of those places on the west coast of Central America—one that's billed as sort of a Hilton in the hinterland. Screens and a thatched roof it had, with as many mosquitoes in as out. All built up on pilings, of course. Somehow I had a feeling someone was watching me as I showered, and sure enough, peering between the random bits of scrap wood that formed what there was of a roof was some sort of a macaw or parrot-type bird. It kept tilting its head one way and another and with

67

that reptilian look they have of having seen everything for millenia, it gave me a towering inferiority complex. Couldn't wait to get a towel around me.

"That was only the beginning. The next day we went out fishing and it was one of those absolutely perfect times, nice breeze, mixed sun, billowy clouds, ocean blue to purple to green. Too good to last. Lucky that I always carry a bare bones surgical kit with me because halfway through the day, one of my buddies hooked a tarpon, a huge thing."

With this, Nick pantomimed the cast and the recoil as the great fish struck then put his fingers over his mouth to indicate the horror as he spoke. "How it happened, I don't know, but the line was around our Indian guide's wrist. The fish made a sudden desperate lunge and the line cut all the soft tissue of the Indian's wrist clear down to the bone—blood vessels, tendons, nerves, the whole blasted bit."

Nick paused for a deep, sighing breath, throwing his hands out in a "what can one do?" gesture, hitched up his bright blue plaid trousers, and continued. "I controlled the bleeding adequately, stitched the skin loosely together, and bandaged him well enough that they could get him into Panama City or wherever they could get him cared for quickly, but we had lost our enthusiasm for fishing out of concern for him.

"Back at our lodge you can bet one of the fellows mixed us each a stiff one, and we were beginning to settle down by dinnertime. After dinner, we sat around listening to the tropical night noises. Under the lodge around the pilings were small scurryings and an occasional squeak of terror. Bats swooped near and low for their evening meal of light-attracted insects and moths. Night comes so suddenly there in the tropics and the light was a bit fitful, the generator being small and temperamental. For that reason it seemed that these Indians just materialized silently in front of us. There were four of them, three men and a woman. After the usual amenities, where neither party really understands the other, one stepped forward. He was the interpreter. 'This man, he chief,' and he indicated an inscrutable middle-aged indigene, clothed in the usual dress of tattered trousers, torn shirt, and makeshift sandals crafted from old tires.

"We nodded and shook hands solemnly. Then the translator went on. 'He thank that you help his friend. Friend son of brother. To thank, he bring you wife to use for night.' Well, of course, I had to do everything but bow and scrape to show my appreciation but without the help of my friends, who could scarcely keep straight faces. I tried to convince the interpreter and the chief that our customs were different and knowing that the injured man would get proper help was enough thanks, etc., etc. Besides, she wasn't my type. They all finally went away after we had given them some cigarettes to soothe any injured dignity anyone might have. I must say that the relief on the woman's face didn't do my ego any more good than the scrutiny of that parrot earlier.

"We were about to turn in when the three men came back again. I never did discover who the third one was. Moral support perhaps. In the chief's arms was a case with a glass top and inside were the most arrestingly beautiful butterflies I had ever seen. I don't know any more about butterflies than about parrots but enough to know that these were probably rare and possibly priceless. They were just like gorgeous pairs of ears. The interpreter made a very gracious if somewhat muddled and mangled speech, and the chief laid the case respectfully in my arms. I made all sorts of grateful noises and hoped the idea got across. Then they left.

"I carried a lantern into my little room and gloated over the beauties in the case. I was so excited it was hard to fall asleep. Next morning before breakfast we took the case out into the daylight to feast our eyes on the iridescence of some of the specimens and the delicacy of shading of some of the others.

"After breakfast we decided that staying in camp wouldn't make our guide recover any faster so the owner sent for another guide and we went out again. Things went better this time. No accidents and the fishing was fabulous. It was nearly dark when we got back and I went right away to my room to look again at my lovely butterflies. They were gone!"

Nick's eyes bugged out of his head, and he let his mouth hang open in dismay. "I was horrified, bereft, scandalized, and hurt. At once I went to the owner and started to raise hell with him, saying someone had stolen my butterflies. He tried to calm me down and poured me a stiff drink, assuring me that he would go at once to see what he could find out, saying that no one ever, ever had anything stolen there and that these particular Indians would starve before they would even take a morsel of food."

"And did he find out what happened to them?" I wanted to know.

"About the time I was going into a real depression over the loss, the owner came back, laughing his head off. He said, 'Remember how the chief offered you his wife for the night?'

" 'Yes, of course. But what has that to do with the butter-flies?'

"The owner nearly choked as he got out the words, 'Well, instead of the woman, the butterflies were for the night.' "

Resolutions

Instead of staying at the restaurant for our after-dinner coffee, we had come back to Ben's place. His bachelor home, modest by Palm Beach standards, was a more enticing spot to end the evening. The second-story mirador was spacious enough to accommodate a collection of rare ferns. Some of his choice orchid plants hung from branches of the huge ironwood and live oak trees. Several of their branches overhung the wrought-iron railing, and the long sprays of pale blossoms fluttered and twirled slowly, mothlike in the light evening breeze.

We were passing the early dusk listening to records of Segovia and Carlos Montoya, the great Spanish classic guitarists, while we exchanged reminiscences of our wrestlings with the Spanish language. I'd learned what I knew by buying some books to help me communicate with the Mexicans who were being cared for in various hospitals in Oregon and California and later with the Puerto Ricans in the Hospital Municipal in Santurce, Puerto Rico. My Spanish was functional, idiomatic, and low on proper grammar. Ben had studied the language at university for several years. His was proper Castilian Spanish and was viewed by Latin Americans with amusement as being rather affected.

He had, he said, as he poured our coffee, promptly dropped the use of the theta when he went to live in South America, not wishing to offend or appear ridiculous to his hosts. With this comment, his mustache twitched in amusement. He often referred to that feature as his "Latin relic."

"Did I ever tell you about my first night in South America?" he asked, as he slid his navy blue blazer from his slightly stooped shoulders and hung it over the back of a nearby chair.

"No. I knew you'd lived there for some years. How did you come to do that?"

"Luck mostly. I was a civil-engineering graduate at a time when they were in great demand and short supply, so in my late twenties I found myself in this capital city in Latin America planning the central water supply and sewage-disposal systems." He ran his hand through his thinning gray hair in memory of the work involved.

I kicked off my high-heeled shoes; my feet were weary after a long day of standing at the operating table, seeing patients in the office, then making hospital rounds. The coffee Ben handed me I perched on the bright tile of a table over which hung a feathery fern.

"Like many people who make a sudden and drastic life change, marriage, new work, or whatever, I thought it would be a good time to take inventory. I'd have a close look at old mental habits and make some resolutions—straighten up my act, as it were. My father, as I've told you, was a minister, and one of his favorite themes was the virtue of humility. It seemed that might serve me well, being so young and in such a responsible position; it might make a good impression. In an alien culture it also seemed a good idea to 'do as the Romans do,' take on protective coloration, if possible."

Pulling over a footstool to better lean back and enjoy the tale, I asked, "About this first night in South America, was it in a hotel?"

Making grandiose gestures in the air, he replied solemnly, "Oh yes, a rather fine one for its time. Of course, that's over thirty years go, so the amenities ran more to personal service than to modern gadgetry. It did have intermittently functioning plumbing, though the water-storage capacity of the hotel tanks wasn't really adequate and, of course, the water was unsafe for drinking. Even for toothbrushing it needed to be chemically treated. The horrible stains on the washbasin were probably from someone's attempts with permanganate—to what end one can't help but wonder."

Ben turned the record over and the volume down while I was flicking a spider over the rail. It had looked down from its home in the fern and seen my coffee cup through its bombsite then drifted down on its silken thread to broaden its world view, just as Ben and I had done each in our own way.

"It was early on a chill evening when I checked into the hotel," he began, "so I unpacked most of my gear, thinking it would probably take a week or so to find a convenient place to live. By the time that task was finished, my hunger was rather acute and it was 9:30, the local dinner hour. I postponed further cleanup until later; after all, I'd had a shave and shower noonish before leaving the ship on which I'd arrived."

While Ben loosened his tie and ran his finger around under his collar, I kicked the footstool out of the way, went to the record player, and turned it off. Much as I enjoyed Segovia, Ben's stories were always worth undivided attention. "Was it a good dinner then?" I asked.

"Of course, and with lots of white-napkin-over-the-arm attentiveness. Beyond that, all I can remember about it was the dessert, the best flan I'd ever tasted. But by this time it was after 10:30 and I was tired, tired, tired and shivering in the unheated corridor on my way to my room and really looking forward to a sound night's sleep." He demonstrated by letting his shoulders sag and his eyelids droop.

After a sip of coffee, his voice was brisk again. "I'd not been back in my room but a minute when there was a knock at the door."

Ben stood up to his full six-foot height to play both characters in pantomime.

"Opening the door, I was surprised to see the *botones*—the bellboy, you know—I'd not rung for him," and Ben gestured as if a door had swung open. His face showed puzzlement.

"Ah, señor" (and with this Ben's eyebrows slid up to a questioning mode and he held his hand palm up in a "would you?" gesture to indicate the bellhop's action), "quiere Usted una señorita?"

"Would I like a señorita? Talk about culture shock. Here I was, a minister's son with the usual moral baggage of chastity and purity and all of that. On the other hand was my resolution to fit into the culture and mores of a place in which I expected to live for some years. Guess what won?" Ben nodded vigorously as if to the *botones* and said, "Sí, sí como no, con mucho gusto. Yes, yes, of course, with great pleasure."

I leaned forward in my chair, eager to hear the culmination of this encounter.

Ben made windmill motions with his expressive hands. "A whirling dervish had nothing on me. To prepare for the arrival of the señorita, in barely over five minutes I'd shaved, showered, put on shaving lotion, and combed my hair. Fresh if travel-wrinkled clothing made me acceptable if not desirable. A quick last-minute glance in the mirror (and with this he slid his hand over his hair and motioned as if to check his necktie) and I opened the door.

"There stood the *botones,* who cocked his head in subservience, saying, 'Aqui está su señorita, señor,' at the same time extending his hands" (pantomimed elegantly by my host). "On them reposed a well-filled hot-water bottle."

74

The Treat

Each of us had our own reasons for being there at the chart desk on the pediatric unit. After saying mass and looking in on the children, Father Dever needed to gather his resources, he said, before braving the adult floors, which at this hour were still mired in bedpans, baths, and breakfasts. His arms were tucked into the full sleeves of his habit, a gesture as habitual as the expression of chronic concern on his ruddy face.

Not being church inclined and too busy to go anyway, I was catching up on my records between dressings and suture removals. Just over a year before, measles had swept through the community, leaving the telltale mark of one cleft lip or palate or both in every eighty-eight white births. That was ten times the usual rate. Depressing.

Jason, the pediatrician, was Jewish, so Sundays didn't obligate him to church; and by making early rounds, he could arrive at the golf course, weather permitting, still in the cooler part of the day.

Selfishly, Father Dever and I regarded Jason, with his expressively mobile features and rabbity eyebrows, as a reliable source of levity to put a little perspective into our endeavors, which at times seemed relatively futile.

This Sunday we needed all the help we could get. The babies were howling, the place smelled, and early rain made grim gray tracks down the windowpanes.

"I'll tell you what's new," he replied to our routine query.

"You may not know how our office is—not candy for the kids on account of cavities, just balloons if they've been good patients. We leave the parents of the older children in our consulting office while we see the children in the examining room. All terribly well thought out and, on the surface, exemplary. Anything to avoid that unexpected fumble that can skew an entire day; parents fainting on the examining-room floor and all of that.

"Anyway, this untidy woman comes in with a blob of nine-year-old boy, a new patient to our practice. To say this kid was dumb or dim would be gross flattery." Jason threw out his hands clumsily and let his mouth hang open to demonstrate. "This kid was stupid with a capital P."

Father Dever nodded and twitched his mouth in a feeble smile. He had apparently encountered the type too often. I couldn't help thinking it must have been soul-dissolving to be glued to the opposite side of a confessional screen from one such, not to mention trying to give meaning to the catechism.

I put a marker in the chart on which I was working and closed it temporarily. "What were they there for?" I wanted to know.

Jason made a grimace and labored on over his characters. "The mother did the talking, belligerent, sort of. 'Johnny's got some trouble. Down there.' She jabbed a finger toward the soiled crotch of his pants."

Jason slid his gaze from side to side as if to avoid reviewing his mental images. "I told her that he might need a little man-type talk and she could wait there in the consulting room while I took Johnny to the examining room. I tried every way of questioning that kid in the book, even the four-, three-, and two-letter words, but no go. That boy was amorphous physically and mentally, and his face didn't have any morph either. How he ever got up off his front paws I don't know. So finally I just gave up on history and examined him. And there it was, a roaring, weeping case of gonorrhea. Finally, desperately, I said to him, 'Where have you been putting that thing?' "

"Pretty basic question," observed Father Dever.

Jason's eyebrows shot up at the comment. "That's it, right down on the ground where the goats can eat it."

"And did you get any answer?" I wanted to know.

"Sort of. Seems as if there was this twelve-year-old girl next door. . . . So Johnny and I went back to his mother. I told her the problem and said he would have to come to the office daily for a shot of penicillin. There's no way you can trust these types to have a prescription filled and take it as directed.

"By this time (and with this admission Jason's eyebrows lowered to an unsteady line), I was exhausted with the whole messy encounter and only looked up perfunctorily as they clumped out the door—that is, until the boy spoke in a voice as expressionless as his face and asked, 'C'n I have a b'loon?' "

One Man's Meat

Nowadays I suppose Rory would be called a "hunk." Back then the word was "heartthrob"; and while we were just platonic friends for old times' sake, it was still a pleasure to be invited for drinks and dinner at his small house near the top of the highest elevation in West Palm Beach.

The late afternoon sun glinted from his copper-colored hair and even redder well-trimmed beard as he bent his tall frame to tend the fire on the grill. A mahoe tree overhung the house and dripped an occasional deep wine–colored flower on the far edge of the patio, accenting the beat of a rather eclectic selection of music—"Puff the Magic Dragon" followed by *Die Fledermaus* and then a group of tangos.

Rory's expressive dark brown eyes flashed with mirth as he related his latest experience with door-to-door salesmen. It always amused me that a person in such a dull job—he was a certified public accountant—would have such a well-honed sense of the ridiculous.

"On Tuesday last," he began, "I'd taken the morning off to clean these wretched mahoe blossoms out of the rain gutters. It's such a trashy tree, but the place would be stark naked without it.

"I'd stopped a minute to stretch and rest my neck, when my eye caught a glimpse of these two intense female types with briefcases and folders. They were clumping purposefully down the street in their clean but very drab outfits—long skirts, long sleeves, and 'sensible' dark laced-up shoes—the whole melancholy missionary bit. You've met this sort, completely joyless, pursuing righteousness with a venom. They are so certain that the quantity of misery they inflict on themselves on this earth will be proportionately rewarded by ecstasy, or some such, in the glorious hereafter. They had a poor waif of about four years of age between them. A heavy bag thumped against the child's long dark dress. You could tell she was weary by the way she dragged her heavy black shoes. There was an uncompromising wide elastic band on her braid. No frivolous ribbons there.

"They couldn't see me, hidden there on the roof behind the branches of the mahoe tree, but they came up to the front step and knocked repeatedly on the door. I'd just finished and wanted desperately to get off the roof and into the house to the bathroom. There was no way I was willing to spend an hour of their time and mine listening to them peddle their version of God. People like that are always so offended and act as if you had personally crucified Christ if you reject their message, no matter how diplomatically. It occurred to me to play their own game so I deepened my voice to intone, 'I am the Lord thy God.' There was a startled squeak from near the front door.

"After a few seconds, I said, 'Thou shalt cast down thy burdens and go forth to preach unto the multitudes, saying unto them, "Dance, rejoice, and make a joyful noise and sing praise unto my name."' After waiting a few seconds and getting nothing but silence from the front step, I tried again. 'Make haste and go now to deck thyself like the bridegroom cometh in gay ribbons and cheerful colors to dance and sing before my face.' I heard frantic scuttling and peered out from my bower to see them running down the middle of the road, pins dropping from their tight hair buns, leaving dun-colored hair streaming down their backs."

By the time Rory finished his story, I was choking with

laughter and wanted to know why he hadn't suggested music with the harp, psaltery, sackbut, and dulcimer.

"Mustn't overdo a good thing, and I did get down to the bathroom forthwith, which was the object of the exercise. Then I gathered up all the religious tracts they had abandoned like worn-out sins and bundled them into a garbage bag, which I sneaked into the dumpster behind Denny's restaurant, where I had lunch on my way back to the office."

Changing the subject radically, he said, "Let's go down to Currie Park for a walk along the lakefront when we finish eating."

That was fine with me for it was a glorious evening and the moon would be up and nearly full by the that time.

We parked about half a block from the park and walked toward the lakefront. Someone nearby had a jasmine in bloom and its scent searched us out now and again on the light breeze. I couldn't help thinking what a seductively romantic setting it was; through the gently waving palms the tips of the wavelets glinted in the moonlight. I would have been content to saunter slowly toward the waterfront, but Rory's stride was purposeful. His thoughts were obviously not on the dreamy attractions of the night.

"I was reading an article in the *Palm Beach Post* about the trouble they're having with the conduit so I wanted to come down here to check out the sewer outfall."

Serendipity

Lois and I were sitting under the locust tree in the late afternoon, drinking lemonade and reminiscing about our time in Africa, my intermittent months and her years there as a teaching missionary and administrator of a small printing shop.

One of the memories we dredged up was that of a game-viewing trip we had made to Sukumi Lodge, with its rustic shelters under the great trees, and the game-viewing drives we had made from that base.

As Lois lifted her lemonade glass, I glanced at her hand to see if she was wearing acrylic fingernails, then asked, "And did you ever get your fingernail back?"

"Oh, that? No, but I saw Sam when I was back in Zimbabwe two months ago. Several of us were staying at Sukumi for a few days, taking a visitor from the States on game-viewing drives, and it was Sam who drove us. He showed me his finger and it had healed nearly perfectly. He said it wasn't tender or anything."

Worrying our minds back through time, we decided it had been eighteen years since Sam had had the accident. He was in his twenties then, thatch haired and already leather skinned from the sun that beat down on the open Land Rover used to drive the guests out to see the animals.

From Sukumi that day we had gone out to watch elephants, giraffes, impalas, and a few zebras, as well as the smaller but no less entertaining congregations of mongeese that ran in and out of the holes in the old termite mounds that were their home. Warthog families, as usual, ran madly across the dry plains at our approach; their stiff tails, held straight up, marked their follow-the-leader progress through the dusty tufts of grass.

Noontime had found us at another bush camp for lunch and a siesta. It was the time just before the rains—dry and oppressively hot with that ominous uncertainty in the air that comes just before the great thunderheads, with their crashing storms, sweep in from the Congo.

We'd finished lunch and had each had a few cans of cold drinks from the cooler, where they had nestled among the ice cubes all morning. Sweaty and sticky, our hair lank and stringing down our necks, we'd stumbled sleepily through the dust to the tents, where we would sleep away a couple of the hottest hours of the day. The animals would be doing likewise so going out to try to see anything would have been unrewarding at that hour.

A loud curse followed by a scream for Flora, my niece, changed the atmosphere from somnolent to electric.

Flora ran back to the main hut and then shouted back for me. Sam knew she had taught at the medical school but hadn't known that it had been bacteriology, physiology, and chemistry and not clinical medicine that had been her forte. As he had been folding up the chairs we had used at lunchtime, he's caught his finger in the metal hinge, cutting through the fingernail and nailbed down to the bone.

Flora jammed his finger into the ice of the cooler as she yelled for me. I had a quick look at the problem and raced back to the tent. Always in my bag is a small bandage scissor, and after quickly removing my bra, I cut the elastic side from it, rescued a clean paper tissue as well, and ran back to the scene of activity. Meanwhile, Lois had come back from her tent to find out what was the cause of the noisy flap.

As much to myself as to Sam, I muttered, "These things are evil injuries. The slightest irregularity in the nailbed after they are healed makes them exquisitely tender every time they are touched. When a man shoves his hand into his pocket or pulls it out, the area can be very painful as it catches on the pocket edge. If I only had a little piece of old X-ray film to use for a splint to keep it smooth and immobile as it heals . . . "

With this, Lois spoke up. "I have an extra artificial fingernail with me. Will it help?"

Serendipity. A wonderful dressing, shaped perfectly, better than X-ray film, and with the even pressure made possible by the elastic from my bra, we couldn't have asked for better.

Sam was to go into Harare the next day for supplies and I made him promise to see about a tetanus shot and have a fresh dressing put on the finger.

Over the years I often wondered if the doctor who saw him was as puzzled about the bandage as I was about something else. What was a lady missionary on a game drive out in the middle of Africa doing with an extra false fingernail?

Constance

When I applied for a secretarial position with the Civil Service back in 1975, I expected a nine-to-five job with the usual holidays. The work would probably be just pounding a typewriter, taking a bit of dictation, and being a general flunky. The whole situation was a matter of financial necessity, which I viewed with resignation and desperation in about equal parts.

Nothing prepared me for the fascination, frustration, pathos, and hilarity that were mine as the secretary to Dr. Mayhew, the director of the forensic laboratory in this jurisdiction. He was a gentleman of the old school but with a wry sense of humor that avoided the trite and tiresome.

The criminal-medicine caseload was escalating by leaps and bounds, and the laboratory was desperately cramped. It had a few poky, ill-equipped spaces in a converted warehouse, which was shared with the local policing unit. Even with additions like encrustations, it was totally inadequate, both in regard to space and equipment. Each year, the legislative body religiously promised new quarters and, just as religiously, appropriated no money for them.

Things came to a head when the vibrations from the firearms section (busy testing a gun from a very sensitive murder case) jiggled the base on which an equally sensitive analyzer rested. It was, at the moment, involved in a determination of equal importance regarding another case. The resulting violent altercation between the personnel of the two departments reached the tabloids, to the acute distress of the director and the mild dismay of the chairman of the legislative committee responsible for oversight. He was too pompous to be much affected, it seemed.

Over the coffee that I fetched to Dr. Mayhew's office, the director and the administrator discussed the dilemma. "Whatever can we do?" groaned the director, twisting the buttons on his lab coat in agitation. "I swear my hair will go white overnight if this keeps on."

I thought it well might as the furrows in his forehead were approaching in depth the thickness of his glasses and gave him the aspect of an anxious owl.

Don Randall, the administrator, shared his view. "We should probably strike now while the iron is hot and the matter in the eye of the public. Such an opportunity may not present itself again very soon. It's unfortunate that the chairman of the oversight committee also chairs the finance committee, which has an immeasurably larger constituency." In his agitation, he spilled both cream and sugar on the table, his lab coat, and trousers. I paper toweled the mess up as best possible without letting it drip off the edge of the table onto my new spectator pumps.

I took my time serving more coffee then brought in my pencil and notebook, not wanting to miss hearing whatever nutty and cockamamie ideas they came up with. In truth, I was devoted to both of them but tended to see them as idealistic little boys trying hard to be good public servants to an unappreciative public. Privately it seemed to me that there was sometimes a certain lack of common sense involved. Often the path of least resistance, like the tortoise, wins the race in the end.

Don Randall, the administrator, had a suggestion. "Let's invite the committee chairman, Edwin Morse, for drinks and lunch and give him a VIP tour so he can really see the problems. That's what we used to do in the service—hog-tie the biggest brass we could get and lay it on thick." He leaned back with his hands behind his head, giving both Dr. Mayhew and I a fine view of the portly expanse of his midriff.

Mayhew snorted. "I noted the emphasis on drinks and think perhaps you may have something there, if not in the tour."

Randall levered his ample self from the chair, turned his little boy grin to both of us, and said, "Fine, I'll go ring him up to see how soon we can get together and leave you and Janet to come up with a good spot for our conspiracy to work its magic."

It didn't take the doctor and I long to settle on a restaurant that had secluded booths, where things could be discussed that aren't usually considered polite mealtime conversation. There would just be the four of us, Edwin Morse, the legislator; Dr. Mayhew, the director; Don Randall, the administrator, and myself, replete with notebook and pencil.

The whole thing was just like a soap opera.

"You see," the director explained to the legislator, "the police are very forceful and keep moving in on our space, then demanding quicker service on their evidence. We need a more up-to-date electron microscope and autoanalyzers, but there is no space for them even if the budget would allow their purchase. You've already seen what havoc the ballistics department can cause. Yet it's not their fault. They really haven't any place that's usable at all. I fear that very soon we, and of course the legislative bodies responsible, will be objects of public jest and ridicule."

"Yes, yes, I see all that." It was evident that legislator Morse was going to "yes" everyone and then once again slide out from under responsibility, though a quick phantom of startled thought was in his eyes when the matter of ridicule was mentioned. Ridicule didn't go with his gray flannel image.

The administrator spoke up. "We insist on giving you a real VIP tour of the facility. All of our analysts are excited about meeting the chairman of the oversight committee."

Seeing the effect of a little flattery on the fellow, the director chimed in, "And I hope to get your autograph for the Eagle Scout in my Scout troop. It would send him into orbit. He'd like to go into law enforcement."

I sniggered to myself. The legislator beamed, and I had to concentrate on my notepad to keep a straight face. It was the first I'd heard of a Scout troop. Must've been a phantom left over from Halloween.

It didn't take a genius to see where this was heading when Dr. Mayhew complained that there was no space to store evidence and some cases were in the works for a long time—like the one of Constance Finian. Everyone knew about that. It had been in the papers off and on for weeks about two years before. Constance was a wealthy widow who had disappeared—poof!—from her summer home in the woods. Police had some suspicions; but without a body or any clues, despite combing the cottage repeatedly, there wasn't much they could do. In the end, though, the expression "Murder will out" proved true.

The disappearance was in very early autumn. Late the following spring, an angler hooked her clothing as he cast in the stream several miles below her cottage, where the river had undercut some large willow roots. That apparently was why she hadn't been found when the stream was dragged in the fall. When brought ashore, it was evident that she was a very well-preserved old woman. She was tanned like a piece of leather and looked like a mummy. The tannic acid from decomposing vegetation and peat upstream had done a perfect job. Interestingly, there was a very deep triangular depression in her head. Her skull had been fractured from a violent blow, but whether it had killed her or just rendered her unconscious so that she drowned in the river was a matter that awaited the coroner's examination.

Again the detective went over the cottage and its environs and found nothing there to account for the injury. Meanwhile, Constance was taking up one of the ten refrigerated drawers in the morgue. She couldn't really be buried until the case was closed. Off and on, when fresh murder victims were brought in, Constance (who really didn't need refrigeration but was kept there for convenience) was evicted from her drawer. Just now she was propped in the corner next to the drawers.

Lunch finished (mine rather spoiled by the presence of notebook and pencil anyway), we all trooped back to the forensic lab. Mr. Morse was fairly well "filled in" as my boss had gestured for the waiter to hurriedly refill the legislator's wine glass while that gentleman was off to the men's room, probably to rearrange the few hairs of his elaborate coiffure.

Our peregrination was weird and wonderful. Dr. Mayhew insisted that Mr. Morse don a stiff, starched white lab coat. That really set the man up. You could see that in his alcoholic haze he fancied himself as an integral, yea verily, an indispensible part of the scientific community. I smiled as we went from area to area, where it was apparent that equipment usually kept put away when not in use had been brought out. Flasks, beakers, and bunsen burners were all bubbling and hissing and flickering away—and in places where even I knew they served no conceivable purpose. Obviously, the director and administrator had briefed everyone very well.

Each one of the technicians and supervisors was presented to Mr. Morse and each gave a highly technical if incomprehensible account of their function, frequently referring to well-known criminal cases. The gentleman was repeatedly thanked for his "abiding interest in the welfare of the law-abiding voters."

Finally, we were just outside of the morgue. Dr. Mayhew's eyes were sparkling with devilishness, but the legislator didn't notice; he was too busy preening himself in his starched clinic coat. He was shown the tiny screened-off hallway where victims were brought on stretchers to be identified by their kinfolk.

"As you can see, this is hardly an adequate area for the purpose, especially if the subject is a floater." The director, administrator, and I crowded in behind and around the poor fellow until he was all but on the empty stretcher.

"A floater?" Mr. Morse's wine-flushed face was suddenly mottled as he struggled to deny what he was trying to think.

"You know," insisted the director a bit impatiently, "the bodies that have been in the water long enough to bloat but not long enough to explode or disintegrate or be eaten."

The color change in the man's face would have shamed a chameleon but there was little time to watch as the director pulled back the curtain and all but shoved the legislator into the refrigerator room with its ten drawers and stainless steel–topped autopsy table. Autopsy knives and saws were ranged on a makeshift shelf that was suspended from the ceiling.

"Here, I'll show you," and the administrator reached for the handle to pull out a drawer.

"No, no, never mind," and with this, Mr. Morse fumbled under the clinic coat to reach for a handkerchief in his pocket.

"Oh, all right. It's just as well. We have an extra leg in with that body anyway. It was pretty badly dismembered, and when they dragged the river for the missing parts, there was an extra arm. We checked with the police across the river and they had an extra leg so we swapped. Only trouble is, they sent us a left leg and we already had one. Some maniac is out there hacking them up faster than those of us along the river can match them up."

I thought it best to get out of the line of fire as the

legislator was looking most unwell. His horrified gaze sought frantically around the room for something on which to fix his mind that would let his stomach and emotions settle. He practically knocked my notebook out of my hand with a jerky uncertain gesture as he pointed to the blackish brown bundle leaning against the wall in the corner.

Airily, Don Randall explained, "Oh, that's just Constance Finian. She's so well preserved we just shove her into the corner when we need her drawer. Would you like to see where her head was crushed in?"

I giggled to myself and allowed as how all this was above and beyond the call of duty, as I knew for a fact that the administrator was no more bloody minded than the legislator.

Mr. Morse bolted from the room, his kerchief covering his face.

The administrator and the director didn't even raid petty cash for the twenty dollars they gave the diener, the morgue attendant, for cleaning up the mess. He was accustomed to worse than that, but I guess his tip was by way of a premature celebration. They knew they'd get the new building this time. Mr. Morse was too much of an egotist to give up the chairmanship of the oversight committee and not strong enough in the stomach to stand another tour of our premises.

The end of the story of Constance did my feminist soul good, it did. One of the detectives was just certain that the answer to the puzzle was in the cottage so he took his lunch in a paper sack and had his wife drop him off there on his day off. When she picked him up that evening, he was all down in the boots—no luck. He told her his troubles. He'd been over the place again and again and could find nothing indoors or out that would make a crushing triangular depression in the skull.

"What about this?" she asked and picked up a kitschy tea-cozy-type quilted cover that was over an old-fashioned sadiron, which served as a doorstop to keep one of the inside doors from banging.

You can imagine the rest. The police called the suspect in and told him they had the murder weapon, with both his fingerprints and Constance's blood on it. Even without the fingerprints, they might have been able to convict him. Only a person who knew the place intimately would be familiar with the sadiron under the cozy and leave it hidden in plain sight as it were.

Idioms

It does seem a bit farfetched, but the Second World War was indirectly responsible for this particular misadventure of Armando's with the English language.

Ordinarily, like many who learn English as a second language, he spoke it more properly than most native-born Americans. It was the idiomatic speech that was his downfall—like the time he referred to someone as a "snake in the mud."

Back to the matter of the war. The chief of my plastic surgery training program, unlike many other plastic surgeons in the area, was beyond the age for military service. As a result, the babies born with cleft lips and palates were referred to his institution from a wide area of the upper Midwest and adjacent Canada. This referral pattern was still in place at the time I was in training there. As a result, we often had one to four or more newborns for cleft-lip closure and five to eight toddlers for palate surgery at any one time.

With this volume, the chief had devised a simpler and more worryfree way of managing these cases than was customary at the time. Those babies who had cleft palates tended to leak all of their fluids back out through the nose as they tried to swallow, so it was common in those days to put down a stomach tube for each feeding. With this method came the attendant possibility of getting it into the lungs and suffocating the infant.

Instead of that, we put a little rice cereal into the formula to thicken it, held the infant upright, and fed them from a whiskey shot glass. It was a little messy but very little came out through the nose and they thrived.

While most surgeons in those days waited until the baby weighed over ten pounds and used a general anesthetic, we operated a day or so after birth if there were no other medical problems. This was done by feeding the infant, giving it a fairly strong sedative, and using local anesthesia. In this way, blood loss was rarely over five cubic centimeters—about a tea-spoon—and the baby was ready for its next regular feeding. It also avoided the prolonged recovery period common in those days of limited choice of general anesthetics as well as their complications.

It was often more difficult to remove the tiny fine sutures from a squiggly neonate than to put them in place. To avoid leaving stitch marks, they needed to be removed in about forty-eight to seventy-two hours. While the wound would be sealed by that time, it was far from healed; and if the seal were disturbed, even a minor separation would result in a wider scar than desirable. For this reason, I resorted to feeding and sedation once again.

Armando had observed this performance several times and had seen me sitting by the dressing room table waiting for sleep to come to the securely restrained infant. While waiting, it was my habit to help things along by patting the wee patient rhythmically on its tummy and talking to it in a low voice. The chant usually went, "There, there, little crumb, you're a nice little baby. There, there, little crumb, you're a nice little baby."

Armando was agreeably impressed with all this and de-cided to try it. Fortunately, it was I, rather than the parents, who peeked into the open dressing room door. The late afternoon sun glinted from the tight dark waves of Armando's hair and put his face in shadow as he bent over the little patient

93

and scrutinized it intently for incipient signs of somnolence. There he sat, patting the infant gently, and intoning over and over, "There, there, you're a crummy little baby."

Dedication

In those days in Bogotá, the very presence of a street lamp was cause for comment. No matter that the scant flickering beam of its evil little eye had to claw its way through the *gurua*. The *gurua*, the thick cloud that squats heavy, wet, and unmoving on the high altiplano, made the uneven streets slimy and the footing perilous. The city had been weighed down with it for days as the miasma hung dead in the air. Between the streets made slick by the *gurua* and the cold, Armando, my husband, was limping more than usual.

We were stumbling from our hotel to a restaurant through a part of downtown Bogotá that had been an elegant residential section years earlier when Armando had lived and gone to school there. The houses had been huge, like the families. Each had three patios: The first was for the señora, a place to cultivate her potted plants and entertain her friends when the weather was favorable. As they had their tea, they could listen to the songs of the birds, whose spacious cages hung in the trees. The middle patio was for the children, with their toys and games. The last one was for the cook, laundress, and maids. On it the clothes could be washed and hung, fowl for dinner killed and plucked, and similar necessary household tasks accomplished. While life may have been cheerful and pleasant inside, these homes were built flush and blind to the street. They resembled forbidding fortresses rather than family sanctuaries.

On this night and in this neighborhood, gentlemen still

wore black vested suits, black hats, and black shoes. Over this elegant but rather depressing attire would be a heavy, white fleecy wool ruana, protection from the cold, wet night air. The dampness of the walkways muffled their footfall, and they would appear as ghosts floating out of the gloom. One such materialized now next to the house on the corner before us. The house itself was more sensed than seen, its vast unlighted bulk menacing in the obscurity.

"This," said Armando, the white hair at his temples glinting silver as he turned his head to speak to me, "is one of the last homes of its kind here. The others, including, as you know, my family home, have been torn down to make way for commercial enterprises. Have I told you the story of Canor Menendez Otero, the handsome, brilliant, and scholarly heir apparent of the family of this house?"

"No, surely I would recall anything about someone with such an unusual name—Canor. Was it a family name?"

"Quién sabe?" he replied, "Who knows? No one ever mentioned it if it was. Anyway," he continued in his pedantically precise English, "I will tell you. You know how, in a small, tight society, in every generation there will be one or two individuals who seem to be anointed by fate and predestined for certain positions in life. As, for instance, my oldest brother, Carlos, who was one such. His interest was in law and government, and when he was barely twenty years old, he was bringing cabinet ministers home for lunch. They would behave as if he had given them a benediction of some kind. *Quién sabe* what he would have accomplished had he not been killed by a hit-and-run driver? Canor was such a person set apart, in some way purer than his peers—in a word, above them. It seems to me that quite often these people are so single-minded and oblivious to all else that they do not perceive dangers, emotional, mental, or physical, that are not central to their obsessive field of interest."

Despite Armndo's steadying arm, my foot slipped on the uneven cobbles of the street, and I lurched heavily against the cold stone of the house. After a few moments, my breath recovered, I inquired, "And Canor, was he also extroverted like your brother Carlos?"

"Ah no, far from it." Armando smiled ruefully and managed a mirthless chuckle. "Very early his scholarly dedication to science was noted, and his teachers remarked with astonishment on the profundity of his knowledge.

"But," he continued, "family and friends were under siege. Canor's two sisters begged to be sent abroad for schooling. They were endlessly annoyed by being courted as surrogates for their brother, whose grandiose prospects were recognized even by the dimmest and most lackluster señoritas. The mothers and even the fathers of seemingly every marriageable girl in Bogotá sought out family friends and relatives, however remote, to implore them to effect some contact with the young man or his parents. I myself recall seeing an ancient, deaf, and bewhiskered crone, who was pointed out to me as the great-great-aunt of Canor, who had also been thus approached. Emotionally, Canor was known as a *palo seco,* a dry stick."

"Given the social scheme of things at that time, he must have spent most of his time dodging around corners," I observed.

"Hardly. Science, particularly anatomy, was his whole life. He seemed deaf and blind to all else. He even managed to ignore his own perforated appendix until he collapsed in the anatomy laboratory.

"The professors at both the Javeriana and Nacional Schools of Medicine vied for him as a student. Each one saw himself as the person who one day could boast of having taught the reowned Canor everything that great man knew. They offered him waivers of fees, free books and equipment, as well as some other more dubious emoluments, in all of which Canor was totally disinterested. He probably didn't even hear their blandishments. He attended the school closer to his home so that less time would be lost traveling to and fro."

Arriving at the Zaguan de los Aguas, "the Vestibule of the Waters," we were seated next to one of the fireplaces toward which I thrust my cold, numb, wet feet. Armando bent toward the fire to read the menu by its light. His deft surgeon's hands leafed through it to find some dish that would remind him of his Colombian heritage and at the same time manage to warm his fingers, which were paper white with chill. This tale promised to be somber and unsettling, and the musical choice of the violinist did nothing to diminish its weight. He was playing that old sad Spanish song of unrequited love, "Dos Cruces" ("Two Crosses"). I sipped my hot mulled rum in an effort to ignore the pain in my bones induced by the altitude and the cold and, as I did so, returned to Armando's epic. "What more do you know of him?"

"He was several years ahead of me in medical school and the first I heard of him directly was the matter of the skeleton."

"The skeleton?"

"Yes. As I've told you, we had to obtain our own. You remember the cemetery here?"

"Oh, yes. When we took flowers to the graves of your parents, Don Carlos and Doña Elvira, we went also to the poor end of the cemetery where the wall is low. You pointed out to me where you'd crouched when you were caught in the crossfire during one of the revolutions."

Meanwhile the violinist had not improved in his choice of selections. Now it was "Sombras" ("Shadows"): "When you have gone, darkness envelopes me."

Armando's eyes shone dark in the firelight as he continued. "That part of the graveyard is the *fossa commune,* where

98

the poor are buried in common graves." He glanced at the nearby tables, which were rather close, and though we spoke in English he said, "When we are back in the hotel, we will find a private corner of the lounge for a nightcap, and I will tell you the rest of the story. We will go by taxi for those few blocks so you will not be chilled again by the weather. What I have to tell you may well do that anyway."

Our dinner finished, Armando handed me into the taxi with typical Latin courtesy. The violinist chose this time to change his pace. The sprightly rhythm of "La Pollera Colorada" ("The Red Petticoat") beat insistently and with a brittle falsity against the ponderous immobility of the night. The notes seemed to shatter against the windows of the taxi to drop their shards in the mud of the gutter.

Seated in a far corner of the lounge of our hotel, Armando bent to massage away the ache in his lame leg as he carried on with the matter of the skeleton.

"Each medical student must go to the caretakers of the graveyard and purchase a complete skeleton from them, which has hopefully been cleaned more or less well. This is no cloak-and-dagger affair. Poor people here realize that if you do not pay for your grave, you are not entitled to have it very long. Nonetheless, most of us were rather diffident about this *negocio* and put it off until the last possible day. Canor, however, was so eager to get on with his studies that he purchased his skeleton in the middle of the preceding term. In that way, the skull would be completely prepared by the time the new term started."

"The skull prepared?"

"Yes. It is filled with dry corn; the foramen magnum, where the spinal cord connects to the brain, is corked firmly; and the whole thing is sunk in a bucket of water. A stone is placed on it to keep it submerged until the swelling corn

99

forces it apart where the bones have grown rather firmly together in adult life."

"I suppose that if it has to be done, whether it is done one day or another makes very little difference."

Armando shook his head. "You would think so, but there is such a superstititious overlay on our Catholicism here that Canor's behavior was a matter of some remark even when it was time for me to secure a skeleton several years later."

"And what else were they saying about him then?"

"Already people spoke about him as if he were dead."

"Already dead?" I asked wonderingly.

"Yes, in one sense of the word it was true." He glanced around to be certain we were not overheard.

"Canor, you see, had an agreement with the doctors who served in the charity wards that he was to be notified of the deaths of patients the study of whose anatomy might further his research. On this particular late evening the deceased was a woman around her midthirties.

"After Canor had been working away over her body for some long time, he became aware that someone was in the room with him. He looked up to see the *diener,* the morgue attendant in charge of cadavers for study. The man opened his mouth to speak when Canor looked up, but Canor was in a bad mood as the answer to his postulated anatomic problem was eluding him so he spoke roughly to the man. 'Get out of here. Go home.' The man tried again to speak, but Canor, enraged, sent the poor fellow scuttling in a volley of curses. The *diener* was the one who told about the episode later. He didn't go home but lurked in the corridor, peering fearfully in from time to time toward the slab on which the cadaver lay.

"Canor, irritated now beyond measure, was tugging, ripping, and tearing impatiently at the tissues rather than approaching them with his usual meticulous dissection. It was late at night when, once again, he sensed the presence of another and glanced up to see a darkish, undefined figure in the door. Resolving not to be diverted again, he turned his attention back to his work in an even more feverish and unrestrained fashion, even throwing instruments on the floor in frustration. Exhausted and angry, he finally raised his head once again to see the figure still in the door. 'You! Who in hell are you and what are you doing here?'

"The meek figure stepped a little forward into the light. It was a very humble *paisano,* turning his hat respectfully in his hands as he ducked his head in subservience.

" 'If it please your grace,' he mumbled sadly, 'when you have finished with my wife, I will take her home so that I may bury her.'

"Canor laid his instruments down on the dissection manual and walked, unseeing, from the door of the room, down the hall, and out into the night. It was as if his humanity, his ability to feel emotion, were born, flowered, and died all in that moment."

"And what did Canor do then?" I asked.

"Nothing really." Armando's voice was low and somber. "He never returned to the medical school, and he never went home. Once in a while someone would stumble over him, drunk and unconscious in a gutter in one of the stinking barrios in the low part of town. The pleas of family and friends went as unheeded as the universal blandishments had been in earlier times.

"No one had seen him or heard of him for months at the time I graduated, so probably he died as he had lived his last months, alone. Even now he probably lies buried, unknown and with scant ceremony, in the *fossa commune.* "

Armando looked beyond the smudgy windowpane and stared, eyes unfocused, into the murk. His voice was low and lifeless, and he murmured as if to himself, "Quién sabe? Who knows? In a few years' time, Canor Menendez Otero may yet return to his beloved anatomy laboratory, this time as a skeleton and skull for the preparation and erudition of another committed scholar."

Informed Consent

Angus Murdock shook his head, and his sandy hair flopped down over hazel eyes that flashed with extreme irritation. His Scottish caution told him that this case could throw his carefully timed retirement plan beyond limbo into purgatory—if you believed in that sort of thing—and, if not, straight to the devil. This would doubtless be a case that would require multiple stages of surgery, with timed waiting between them for circulation and healing to establish itself in flaps and grafts.

Worse still, in the end the patient might be healed but look a mess. As the only one of his specialty in the area who dealt with complex reconstructive problems, he did not see how he could refuse the case, especially as it had been referred by his fishing buddy, Jim Crockett.

Swiveling his chair to put his brogan-clad feet up on the wastebasket, he stretched his lanky frame back, hands behind his head, and thought about it. He had seen several of these Vietnamese women who had had silicone injections into their breasts. Temporarily it might make them more attractive to the GIs, Angus supposed. Unfortunately, the material was usually adulterated with irritants to set up scar formation so that it wouldn't drift. Once he had had some of it analyzed and was horrified to learn that the adulterant had been crankcase oil.

Angus could just see his little fishing shack on Oregon's Rogue River evaporate into the mists of the indefinite future.

With it went the trip to the north country he and Jim had planned in order to try their luck for muskelunge. "Jim has really fouled my line this time," he muttered crossly to himself.

The irony of the situation didn't escape Angus. He rather disliked his accountant on a personal basis. The fellow was a rather prissy little man, with unevenly and inexpertly applied hair dye that fluoresced in some lights. Being downwind of him was suffocating. Surely only a bubbling punch bowl of all the perfumes on a Woolworth counter could manage such an effect. Nonetheless, the man had told Angus explicitly how to roll over his profit-sharing and pension trust plans to the best tax advantage. Now the whole deftly arranged early retirement scheme was about to be sabotaged by a teaspoon of crankcase oil, castor oil, or some other revolting substance. In his mind's eye, he could visualize the draining wounds, feel the large knots in the axillae, and smell the sickish sweet odor of the chronically infected wound.

A potentially more serious problem was the current malpractice crisis. At last week's symposium the newest wrinkle had been thoroughly discussed. The patient would claim a lack of fully informed consent. No matter how simply worded the consent form might be or how lengthy the explanation, a patient could say they "never really understood all of that." It was unfortunate that the law assumed that all patients were mentally able and intellectually and emotionally willing to understand. Here would be a patient whose condition did not permit a good result. Simple healing was the best for which anyone could hope. She probably didn't understand English either.

"Ah, well." Angus shrugged his shoulders out of the corduroy jacket with its worn leather elbow patches, and slid into a starched white clinic coat. His Scottish Presbyterian Bible training came to his aid. "Every day is sufficient unto the evil thereof." He would simply do the best he could and hope he could bring some understanding of the extent of the problem to the patient. He would be seeing her at the end of the day, so if the visit dragged on, as it well might, it wouldn't put his office schedule behind. He would worry about hospital rounds later.

At 4:30 Miss Landers showed a young couple into his office, handed him the chart, and said, "Mrs. Hutchinson to see you with her husband, Corporal Hutchinson, to translate for her."

Doctor Murdock shook hands with each of them and indicated chairs across from his desk. He turned to the petite lady, noting her thinness and the lack of luster in her big dark eyes as she glanced nervously about. "I understand you have a breast problem, Mrs. Hutchinson."

Her wary glance turned to her big, broad-faced, uni-formed husband, who leaned forward. "She don't speak much English, Doc."

"Well then, can you tell me how long ago this problem began?"

In answer to a question in her own language, the little lady murmured a few words to her husband.

"About four years ago she had some injections. I didn't know her then. Only met her two and a half years ago."

Angus pursed his upper lip with its mustache thought-fully between his forefingers. "How many injections did she have and were they done by the same person?"

As she and the corporal exchanged a few words, Angus felt Mrs. Hutchinson was aging, diminishing and shriveling under his very gaze. She nervously rubbed the dry skin of her arms while the corporal spoke. "About three injections each side, a different person each time. She didn't have any prob-lems when I first knew her—well, maybe a little lumpi-ness—but she never complained and they looked all right."

Doctor Murdock took a deep breath and considered the

105

problem. The possibility of six adulterating substances might not make any difference in the breast area proper, but who was to know how toxic some of the witches' brew could be to her kidneys or liver if it had been picked up by the circulation?

A full fifty minutes later he had extracted as much general medical information as could be gleaned through an interpreter who was obviously very concerned and willing but none too fluent in his wife's language. He had also done a complete physical examination and brought the couple back into his consulting office.

Sighing deeply, he said, "I'll give it to you straight, Corporal Hutchinson. This is very serious and will need several stages of surgery, with hospital care in between. Will your benefits permit this to be done in the military hospital in the next state? It will be very costly."

"Naw, Doc," the corporal shook his head. "Nobody there could understand her. I'm all my wife's got except for a Vietnamese girlfriend whose husband is a buddy of mine. She speaks a little more English than my wife. The government may pay something toward her care here, and I've lined up a part-time moonlighting job as a bartender. It pays good but it may take me awhile to pay off everything."

Angus Murdock admired the way the big, slow-spoken fellow shouldered the responsibilities of an open-ended problem and felt that with such an example he could do no less.

"Very well. It is most important that your wife understand everything that will happen or could happen. We will do some X rays and laboratory studies to see if any infection or poison has spread to Mrs. Hutchinson's liver, kidneys, or anywhere else. If it has not, there is still a chance that this could happen during treatment. She could become permanently ill through the spread of the infection or even die, though that is unlikely.

"All of this must be removed down to the ribs." Angus traced his finger on her chest to show the extent of the surgery. "After we are sure the infection is gone, we will take skin—probably from there and there (pointing to her thighs and buttocks)—to put on the raw places. There will be light patches and some scarring where we take the skin. The skin we put on her chest will look like patches. She is much too thin and ill to consider trying to make new breast mounds. Perhaps if she were to get fat some day . . . " he let the sentence dangle. With luck he would have done his duty and be long gone by then, and someone else could face that hurdle. That would be a couple of years away at least, if he estimated her chronic illness accurately.

"Now." His light hazel eyes looked straight and carefully first at Mrs. Hutchinson then at her husband. "It is most important that the patient understand each of these problems in detail and ask any questions there may be. Will you please tell your wife, word for word, as best you can, what I have said."

Corporal Hutchinson turned to his wife and put his arm protectively over her shoulder. She looked up at him, her expression a mixture of trust and fear.

"Doctor say," the corporal summed the whole into four succinct words, "titty may fall off."

Birth Control

The three of us were sitting around the campfire at Mana Pools in Zimbabwe. We were eating hash made from kudu, potato, and onion and exchanging medical experiences as varied as the ingredients in the hash.

Conversation was quiet and fitful as we had to listen for elephants. The camp was unfenced, and at this time of year they came, usually at night, to feast on the pods of the great acacia trees. They had also developed a taste for citrus fruit and had been known to demolish tents and break into vehicles for oranges.

Marnie was a nurse from one of the mission hospitals a good ways out in the *bundu* from Karoi over road that seemed bumpier than the terrain around it. We had been helping her with one of her child and maternal-health clinics on the way to the campground. Weighing screaming, weeping, little black *totos*, whose pupils were rimmed white with terror, was old hat to Marnie. She could sling the rope that held the scale over a tree branch as readily as a skilled cowboy could rope a steer. It was familiar stuff also to my niece, Flora, who had worked with the missions and taught in the medical school in Salisbury (called Harare now that Southern Rhodesia had become Zimbabwe).

"Did I tell you," Marnie wanted to know, "about one of my family-planning failures at the clinic over west of the mission? I was there just last week. I'd been there four months before with a goodly quantity of Western European government-supplied condoms to give to couples when the woman couldn't tolerate the side effects of birth-control pills. Of course the men don't come to the clinics, so our instructions had to be conveyed to them through the women."

Knowing the attitudes of the local African males toward childbearing, Flora asked what success this condom project had had, considering that many of the men would probably not permit their wives to take the pill. In this area, children were considered an economic asset as much as proof of a man's virility.

Marnie had been in Africa long enough to know she couldn't win them all and answered, "Success? Mixed. Like in everything else. If all goes well, you never really know about it, but when things go wrong . . . "

"I take it something went wrong," Flora prodded.

"Giving instructions to these ladies on the use of a condom was supposed to be easy—so the program doctor told us. He, of course, was European and had never lived or worked in the bush. That probably accounted for the fact that the instructions were more on the lines of euphemism than realism. He showed us how to demonstrate the application of a condom by pulling it down over our thumb, leaving some space at the end, etc., etc. Using the local terminologies as best possible, without being offensive to my clientele, I had done as he said. I went back last week to that clinic to find one of the women pregnant."

"Didn't you and your husband use the condoms I gave you?"

"Oh yes, madam, just exactly as you said and showed me, but my husband says he really can't understand how wearing that thing on his thumb will keep me from getting pregnant."

Jade

Psychiatrists' offices tended to be personality neutral in Bud McClintock's opinion and this gave an added fillip to his sleuthing. "I might as well be a Peeping Tom or voyeur of some kind, looking about another physician's office in his absence. Nothing here to indicate why he has been so insistent in asking about my vacation plans. No pictures of big fish or golf courses."

His colleague, Luke Brauer, had excused himself for a few moments to give direction to the secretary. Bud occupied the time with a swift mental dismissal of the bookcase with its medical books and journals, the leather easy chairs, the unremarkable drapes and carpet.

Ah, here was the nugget. On one shelf was a solitary item—an exquisite, delicate jade frame, small. It was a double frame. On one side were Oriental characters (very fine calligraphy, Bud thought). The opposite side of the frame displayed a traditional wedding announcement.

> Mr. Donald Martin
> announces the wedding of his sister
> Miss Lynn Martin
> to
> Mr. Paul Cheng
> in
> Hong Kong
> July 11, 1970

Fascinating, Bud thought, but certainly nothing to relate to persistent queries about his vacation time.

He lifted a matching frame from the unobstrusive desk. It held two pictures of a Eurasian girl about two and a half years old. One was a professional photograph, the child neatly dressed and seated on a low cushion with a kitten in her lap. The other was a snapshot. She was in a pair of dirty sneakers and filthy shorts, a pail of sand and a shovel beside her as she grubbed near the surf on a beach. Bud had never seen a picture of a child with such a luminous smile.

Here was the key to Luke's psyche, he thought, Luke, the physician who had seemingly led a life of monstrous monotony since the death of his much-loved wife. Bud replaced the pictures on the desk just before Luke reentered the room.

"Sorry to leave you, but you now how it is to shift scheduling. We have time for a drink before the meeting. Would you like it here or in the lounge across the street?"

"Here, if you'll tell me the story of the pictures in the jade frames. There aren't enough clues to piece together, and I sense a curious tale—perhaps related to our specialty?"

Luke bent to open a disguised refrigerator for ice as he spoke. "Yes, and although the help I gave was inadvertent, it made my entire professional life worth the effort, my personal life as well."

"A strong statement from one of a fraternity given to bland, noncommittal remarks. Begin at the beginning and we'll finish after the meeting." Bud lifted his glass. "Here's to your lifetime number-one success."

Luke reached to the bookshelf for a well-worn book, which opened automatically to the place where a photograph was kept. Handing it to Bud, he began.

"Jonas called me one day and asked me to see a patient as soon as possible. He's not the type to cry wolf, so I told him to have the patient come by at the end of office hours. As an afterthought, I asked for the name and roughly the nature of her problem. He said, 'Her name is Lynn. Problem? Beauty.'

"When she came into the office, I nearly gasped. Despite her downcast aspect, she was the most beautiful creature I had ever seen. In that dragging voice depressed patients can have, she said simply, 'I'm Lynn from the plastic surgeon's office. I feel that something in the core of me is fragmenting and suicide seems, well, reasonable.' "

Luke sipped at his drink. "I must tell you that I saw this patient only twice in my life. That first time she was the saddest sane person and the second time the happiest—almost luminous. That photograph is of her in her wedding gown."

Bud held the photograph for some minutes, his drink forgotten. "God, she's exquisite, more than beautiful." The classic high mandarin neckline, plain long sleeves, and lightly fitted dress enhanced her appearance rather than competing for attention as he thought bridal gowns rather tended to do. Light golden brown hair framed a face, whose dark hazel eyes bespoke great happiness and contentment.

Bud shifted in his chair and handed back the photograph. "There's something vaguely familiar though not with this radiant expression. Should I recognize her?"

Luke put the picture away in its book. "Possibly. A few years before this was taken she modeled diamonds and emeralds for the world's premier jeweler. She may have done a little other modeling but not much I think."

Bud pondered that a moment. "Given the money made by a top model and her beauty, one would think, in the parlance of our youth, that she would have 'had it made.' Whatever was she doing in a shrink's office?"

Luke took the empty glasses to the secretary's nook and grabbed up his jacket. "That's the second installent. It comes after the meeting."

Bud didn't really hear the speaker. He was preoccupied

with Luke's story and mused to himself that there was probably a great deal more to it than simply a pretty girl marrying a Chinese fellow on the other side of the world.

After making the obligatory polite noises to the other attendees following the meeting, he took Luke's arm. "I know a place for dinner where the service is so slow we can finish your story of the lovely lady, even if she's eighty years old now.

"She isn't anymore." Luke's voice was low.

Both fell silent as they picked up menus. Bud felt Luke was reliving a bittersweet memory. Had he loved the girl?

Their orders in and the waitress departed, Luke enlisted his fellow psychiatrist's knowledge. "It seemed to me she was very close to that state of emotional soddenness when she wouldn't be able to communicate at all. Her two sentences sounded like a phonograph record slowing down to a stop."

Bud nodded and prodded him. "So you tried to make a lucky strike on something that would elevate her mood enough to start her talking."

"Naturally. I asked her to start with her childhood, and I'll try to tell you the story, more or less in her own words.

" 'My childhood? The best part of life. My parents were older than most when I was born, and Donald came along eighteen months later. We were just two of about a dozen untidy towheads, who spent the days with mud pies, hopscotch, marbles, butterfly catching, and later hide and seek in the long twilight. Grade school was fine too; in a small town, schoolteachers really knew everyone and cared about each child.' "

While the waitress wielded the peppermill over his salad, Bud was pensive. "It surely doesn't sound like one of those horribly deprived childhoods that all but leave a nasty tattoo on the soul."

"No, but when I asked about adolescence, it all came tumbling out as if she were living it over again.

" 'You know how kids are,' she said. 'One day just kids and the next day all elbows, knees, pimples, lank oily hair, and braces on their teeth? Only that didn't happen to me. It seemed that just overnight I was like I am now, only ten years younger. Every night I'd pray to wake up with lop ears or crooked teeth or something so the other girls would include me in their tight little whisperng clusters. You wouldn't believe the silence that would greet me when I walked into the girls' lounge, where they were chattering and giggling together about hairdos, face lotions, orthodontists, and boys. . . .

" 'Finally, I cornered the boldest one and asked if I had leprosy or something. She just told me, in very vulgar language, to shove off. They didn't want me near them or their boyfriends or anyone who might be a boyfriend in the future. No matter how hard I tried, only one girl would be friendly to me—Rosa. Her folks were Mexican, and she was really nice. The other girls wouldn't have anything to do with her either.' "

Luke put his fork down. "When I asked how long that friendship lasted, her eyes filled with tears as she answered, 'Not long. I had to run through a thorn hedge to get away from her uncle. I just couldn't tell her why I wouldn't come to her house anymore, so she called me a snotty gringo and that was that.' "

Buttering a bit of dinner roll, which he chewed slowly, Bud looked up at Luke. "Not much point in asking about boys, is there?"

Luke shook his head. "Not much. Those who weren't fenced away by other girls or who weren't what she called 'the grope-and-grapple gang' were so shy they were intimidated by a plain 'Hello.' They turned red in the face and fled."

Luke scanned the dessert menu then said, "I guess one of the most traumatic things that happened was at the senior dance. Some boy cut in on Lynn's brother, who'd escorted her. The boy's girlfriend ran screaming across the dance floor, shoved her boyfriend away, slapped Lynn's face, ripped her dress from her shoulder, and yelled, 'Greedy bitch' at her."

"Horrible," muttered Bud, as he shook his head both at the story and the offer of dessert.

"Anyway, that episode was followed shortly by her father's death, and the discovery of her mother's illness made the move to the city welcome. She juggled modeling jewelry, part-time classes at a girls' school, and caring for her mother (with her brother's help) fairly well. After her mother's death, she even had three gentlemen friends, as well as encounters with the 'pat-and-pounce posse.' "

"And how did the romances go?" queried Bud, between sips of coffee.

A rueful smile crossed Luke's face. "The first was very attentive and gentlemanly, busy camouflaging his homosexuality. The second, according to Lynn, 'wore me on his arm the same way a newly rich woman wears an ostentatiously vulgar piece of jewelry.'

"The last was such a sorry story she could hardly speak about it and finally sat in a lumpy little heap, sobbing quietly. When she gathered herself together enough to talk, she said, 'By this time I realized that the great happiness my parents had in each other and their children might well pass me by. Panicky, I did something so selfish that it will haunt me until I die.'

Luke folded his napkin and continued in Lynn's words. " 'It seemed maybe, if someone couldn't see me, just maybe . . . and it was easy to be a volunteer at the school for the blind. There was a young man there . . . oh, I wasn't in love with him, but he was so nice. His students loved him for his sense of humor, and somehow he made them feel that blindness was an inconvenience, a nuisance, not a terrible handicap. I'd fix dinner for us and we'd go dancing. I began to feel abashed about making such a great thing of "my problem," never mentioning it to him of course.' "

Luke was quiet, while Bud signed the Visa card, and then went on. "She started to cry again, not sobbing, just tears plopping down on her blouse as she explained. 'He feels differently now and very bitter. His sighted friends thought it great fun to make up stories about how I was behaving just because he couldn't see. I tried to tell him they were lying and teasing, but we each ended up sour and disconsolate, he because he felt he couldn't trust me and I because he believed his buddies instead of me. That's when the depression started to be a real problem. Only my brother, my job, and my hobby kept me somewhat stable.' "

As they stood to leave the table, Bud asked, "What was she doing?"

"Working at a day-care center at a financial loss, which she could afford to do. Loving other people's children was a poor third to her own, she told me, but it was good therapy for a naturally affectionate, nurturing person."

Bud paused outside the restaurant door to accustom his eyes to the dark. "And what about her brother?"

Luke appreciatively sniffed the air from which a light rain had laid the dust, then led the way down the sidewalk. "Always supportive. Two things Donald did at this juncture were great. First, he took karate lessons and came home to teach Lynn. She told me his remark was a grim, 'I figure you'll need this when I leave, Sis.' Then one day he and his girlfriend took her to a showing of jade carvings at an art gallery. They had been done by an ancient native woman living in Vancouver."

Bud stepped off the curb to cross the street. "And what did she do about that?"

Luke grunted. "Let it rescue her temporarily." She put it to me this way, 'I'd never seen anything so soft and lovely. Jade is warm and has a soul. It's not harsh and brittle like the diamonds and emeralds I'd been modeling.' She made arrangements to spend her vacation with the old lady to learn the rudiments of the craft and something of ivory carving as well. I'll show you her last work when we get back to the office for our nightcap."

"And Jonas," queried Bud, "where does he fit in?"

"Her depression slowly deepened after Donald married and moved to Dallas, so in one of her more dismal moods she asked Jonas to put a hump on her nose."

Bud blurted a shocked and startled, "No!"

"She said he was very nice about the request and studied her face seriously for some time. Then he told her that quite apart from the fact that it would do his reputation no good, he felt it would simply change her from lovely to elegant and she would be less approachable. When I asked how she came to see me, she managed a wisp of a smile."

" 'He sat quietly for a few minutes,' she told me, 'apparently running things through in his mind, how to phrase what he wanted to say without being flippant or offensive. Finally, Dr. Jonas leaned across his desk and said, "I'd like you to talk to Dr. Brauer. He's a bit more than a psychiatrist. He's, well, a bit unstructured in some of his ideas. His thinking lacks constricting walls. That's badly put, I know, but he thinks of things between inventive and conniving that wouldn't occur to more buttoned-down types.' "

Bud laughed out loud as they entered the door of the office building. "I don't know if that flatters you professionally and damns you personally or the other way around."

Luke nodded his head. "Either way, it didn't give me any ideas, but an odd thing happened. As a way of terminating an interview that had certainly led nowhere, I said, as kindly as possible, that I guessed her best hope was to find someone with a different idea of beauty."

"And what was her response to that?" asked Bud, as he indicated the Drambuie bottle.

"She looked at me, stood up, shook hands firmly, and said, 'Thank you for your time, Dr. Brauer. May I keep in touch?' She seemed to have gleaned some comfort or resolve from the time we'd spent talking.

"I thought of her now and then and wondered what had happened. Finally, I had my secretary ring Lynn's phone number only to get a recorded, 'That number is no longer in service.' "

Luke mulled over the bottles and finally settled on a small brandy then continued. "After about four months a letter arrived from Hong Kong. She was, she wrote, in need of a surrogate parent and very delicately indicated that she would be happy to pay my professional fee. Enclosed from the business personals of a dual-language newspaper was a want ad: '*Seeking person with knowledge and interest in ivory and jade carving and jade mining.*' She had enclosed her phone number with the letter, so I checked the time zone and called her."

"Why the ad?" Bud lifted his brows.

"That's what I asked after pleasantries were exchanged and I'd told her my fee would be the satisfaction gained from a 'far out' case. She laughed, a great mood change from our office conversation.

" 'I reasoned thus,' she told me. 'Carvers of jade and ivory here will probably be Orientals. It is unlikely that a woman or an old man would be interested in the mining aspects, especially since the best jade now is coming from British Columbia and Alaska, particularly a mine in Alaska above the Arctic Circle.' "

"Teasing her a little, I wanted to know what else her reasoning had told her to do. Her tone was serious. 'I've hired a rather late-middle-aged lady, who was a fugitive from the mainland. She runs the household and is teaching me basic

118

Chinese manners and customs, together with some of the language.' "

Bud muttered, "Well, if nothing else, she's too busy to be introspecting."

"That's true, but she'd done enough of that to ask if I thought she had been too bold. It seemed to me she had not, by our standards, but I recommended she take further advice from her Chinese mentor. We closed the conversation on that note, and she agreed to keep me posted on her progress."

Bud sipped at his Drambuie. "This is quite a cliff-hanging soap opera. My practice is certainly dull and pedestrian in comparison."

"Agreed," Luke nodded, "and it gets more intricate. Some several months later, a long, glowingly happy letter arrived. One Paul Cheng had answered the ad. He was, she reported, a truly fine man and a connoisseur of narwhal and walrus ivory, as well as a jade carver of some repute. As a result of a difficult birth (which had cost the life of his mother), he had seizures that were not completely controllable by medication. For that reason he needed someone with him when he traveled, and though he had wanted to go to North America for materials, as yet it had not been possible. And best of all, he thought his older sister was the ideal of beauty.

"Lynn described Melinda Cheng as being absolutely lovely, with jet black hair, ivory skin, and almond eyes. Apparently, when she was in a room, all eyes were on her. Lynn found her a delightful person, who had managed to avoid the bind that she, Lynn, had been unable to escape. Lynn said she thought perhaps Melinda's personality was better integrated or perhaps Chinese men were more formal in their approach to women. Anyway, for the time she was very happy and said that I might hear from Paul before long."

"And why would *you* hear from him?" Bud wanted to know, as he put his feet up on a hassock.

119

"To my surprise," Luke replied, "age may be more important than relationship, at least in some Oriental families. In just a few days, a rather formal letter arrived from Paul Cheng, requesting my permission to propose marriage to Lynn. Naturally, I felt this placed me in a rather awkward position, so I called her brother, Donald, who whooped with laughter. He'd already heard from Lynn and was so pleased he said he didn't care whether the letter was addressed to me, the devil, or the man in the moon."

Bud had another sip of his Drambuie. "What happened next?"

"Some months later, Donald, his pregnant wife, and I went together to Hong Kong for the wedding. I gave the bride away, Donald was best man, and Melinda Cheng, Paul's sister, was maid of honor. The wedding was Western, after a fashion, but with enough of the Chinese traditions to make it interesting—even numbers of flowers in the arrangements and so on."

Luke topped up the drinks and continued. "In a few months, Lynn wrote that she was expecting, and they would like me to be godfather. I phoned at once with congratulations and acceptance. You'd be surprised how much enjoyment it gave this rather desiccated widower to be a cherished part of a family."

"So did you go for the christening, bell ringing, or whatever they have?"

"No," Luke sighed. "I planned to, but a bad case of flu didn't seem a gracious gift so I stayed here and was hospitalized eventually."

"I remember." Bud nodded his head. "You were on the fifth floor, quite ill."

"Not so much so, but alone at home one doesn't even have a passable chance at a quick recovery. I'm still indebted to you for offering to cover emergency calls from my patients.

Your kindness prompted my inquiry about your vacation plans."

"Oh, that, no problem." Bud brushed off the thanks and picked up the child's picture. "Did you ever get to see the baby then?"

"Oh yes. Each of the next two years when Lynn and Paul went to the Arctic for jade and ivory, Melinda brought her to the States. We were all together with Donald's family at the beach."

Luke reached into his pocket to draw out a small jewel box. He opened it and handed Bud a jade ring with a delicate tracery carving. "This is Lynn's last work. Do you like it?"

Bud examined the ring with great interest. "It's exquisite, but isn't it too big for the little girl?"

"It isn't for my daughter," said Luke, shifting in his chair so his face was out of the light.

"Your daughter!" Bud stammered, "But I thought . . . "

"Lynn and Paul were killed in a light-plane crash on the way to a jade mine about six months ago. I've adopted their child. I would like you to be the best man at my wedding in Hong Kong when I give this ring to Melinda Cheng."